D0934947

ASHAMED TO DIE

ASHAMED TO DIE

Silence, Denial, and the
AIDS Epidemic in the South

ANDREW J. SKERRITT

Lawrence Hill Books

Chicago

EMMET O'NEAL LIBRARY
50 OAK STREET
MOUNTAIN BROOK, AL 35213

616.9792

Copyright © 2011 by Andrew J. Skerritt
All rights reserved
Published by Lawrence Hill Books
An imprint of Chicago Review Press, Incorporated
814 North Franklin Street
Chicago, Illinois 60610
ISBN 978-1-56976-814-3

Library of Congress Cataloging-in-Publication Data
Skerritt, Andrew J.
   Ashamed to die : silence, denial, and the AIDS epidemic in the South / Andrew J.
Skerritt.
       p. cm.
   Summary: "By focusing on a small town in South Carolina, this study of the HIV/
AIDS crisis in the South reveals the hard truths of an ongoing and complex issue. Skerritt contends that the United States has failed to adequately address the threat of HIV
and AIDS in communities of color and that taboos about love, race, and sexuality-
combined with Southern conservatism, white privilege, and black oppression-continue
to create an unacceptable death toll. The heartbreak of America's failure comes alive
through case studies of individuals such as Carolyn, a wild child whose rebellion coincided with the advent of AIDS, and Nita, a young woman searching for love and
trapped in an abusive relationship. The results are most visible at the town's segregated
burial ground where dozens of young black men and women who have died from
AIDS are laid to rest. Not only a call to action and awareness, this is a true story of how
persons of faith, enduring love, and limitless forgiveness can inspire others by serving
as guides for poor communities facing a public health threat burdened with conflicting
moral and social conventions"—Provided by publisher.
   Includes index.
   ISBN 978-1-56976-814-3 (hardback)
   1. AIDS (Disease)--Southern States. 2. African Americans--Diseases--Southern
States. 3. Social medicine--Southern States. I. Title.
   RA643.84.S85S54 2011
   362.196'979200975--dc23
                              2011016724

Interior design: PerfecType, Nashville, TN

Printed in the United States of America
5 4 3 2 1

EMMET O'NEAL LIBRARY
50 OAK STREET
MOUNTAIN BROOK, AL 35213

DEDICATION

—⊶⊷—

To my grandmother, Peggy Skerritt, who first
taught me the importance of writing and letters; to my wife
and children, whose steadfast support kept me awake past too
many midnights; to Audra, my agent, who believed in this project
from the moment she discovered it; to the Reverend Patricia Starr;
and to the memory of Carolyn, Nita, Tracy, Robbie, Girard,
and the others who entrusted me with their stories.

CONTENTS

ACKNOWLEDGMENTS

This book would not have been possible without the
generous cooperation of too many people to mention.
Seldom did anyone refuse an opportunity to tell his or her story.
I am eternally grateful to Patricia Ann Starr, Linda Ashley,
Margaret Jenkins, Chris Blanton, Rebecca Melton, Barbara Dixon,
Charles White, and doctors Robert Ball, Phil Lackey, Craig Charles,
and Michael Watson. Fate conspired to make the fight against
HIV and AIDS part of their lifework. Again, thanks.

PROLOGUE

One fall day in 2000, I walked into a church hall in Rock Hill, South Carolina, and took my seat among a group of white mothers and daughters. The guest speaker was Reverend Patricia Ann Starr, who had gained local notoriety for her work with people living with acquired immune deficiency syndrome (AIDS). Reverend Starr was dark-skinned, heavyset, and carried herself like a woman who had spent a lifetime thinking she wasn't much to look at. She had Jheri curls and wore no makeup or jewelry—the unadorned appearance of a traditional woman of faith. At the time, she hadn't yet turned forty, but a casual observer could have easily mistaken her for a fifty-year-old woman. The burdens of life seemed to rest squarely on her shoulders. Starr had recently been appointed pastor of True Word of God Fire Baptized Holiness Church, a small evangelical congregation in York, South Carolina. Each week, she wrestled with how to teach her black, rural congregants to practice their faith in an increasingly complex and secular world. Reverend Starr was largely self-taught. She quit Clover High School during her freshman year to care for her ailing mother, Annie Mae Pegram. She became a mother at fifteen and a wife at sixteen. Although Starr promised her mother she would return to school to earn her GED, she never did. A childhood of poverty, sickness, shame, disappointment, and death provided all the education Starr would ever need. Surprisingly, she escaped the bitterness and cynicism that so often comes from a hard life. That qualified her for a mission of redemption and grace. But in the 1990s, fate mandated a new, more urgent message beyond the call to rescue souls from hell and damnation.

That Saturday morning, Starr told those mothers and daughters about AIDS, a silent epidemic killing men and women in her predominantly black neighborhood in Clover, a small textile town forty minutes south of Charlotte, North Carolina.

Starr spoke about people who used sex for currency and escape, the cheapest means toward a sad end. All of the sex and drugs couldn't mask the pain that came from the poverty, childhood abuse, domestic violence, unemployment, and hopelessness that too often dominated the streets and neighborhoods of small southern towns. She sought to warn the young women seated before her that their social status wouldn't inoculate them from the dangers of unprotected sex.

Less than ten years earlier, Starr had only heard of AIDS as a disease afflicting homosexual men in major cities. As a person of deep religious faith, she initially found it hard to sympathize with those who suffered after "violating God's laws." Then her sister Carolyn, the wild child of the family, was diagnosed with the human immunodeficiency virus, HIV. As Carolyn careened from one health emergency to the next, Starr learned that others in her neighborhood were also infected with HIV/AIDS, an illness that neutralizes the body's immune system and renders its host vulnerable to deadly, opportunistic infections. For Carolyn and others living with AIDS, a common cold became a potentially life-threatening illness. Starr's attempts to help her sister opened doors to her starting a food pantry, which in turn led her to providing comfort and daily support to her neighbors dying of AIDS.

On that Saturday in Rock Hill, South Carolina, Reverend Starr delivered a simple but hyperbolic message to the small group. "It doesn't matter who you're with. If you take chances and have unprotected sex, it—AIDS— is going to get you."

Reverend Starr spoke for about an hour. Hush ruled the huge room as the women and girls sat in silent disbelief. Nothing in their experience could have prepared them for the unlikely story they were hearing. Seated at the back of the room, pen and notepad in hand, I listened spellbound.

After Starr ended her speech, I introduced myself, took her phone number, and returned to the newsroom to research old clips and the electronic library. Her name hadn't graced the pages of the *Rock Hill Herald*—not for birth announcements, obituaries, or police blotter items. I was determined to change that. It would be months before my story finally appeared, just in time for World AIDS Day 2000. Titled "AIDS in a Small Town," the story was accompanied by a photograph of Starr standing in front of her home with her niece Tracy as she spoke to a group of young men from the neighborhood. What the caption didn't say (and I didn't know at that time) was that Tracy, like her aunt Carolyn, was HIV positive. The story told of how AIDS stalked the streets, especially in the predominantly black sections of Clover, and of the silence and denial that made a lethal illness even more deadly.

After that initial foray, I became an advocate for public awareness. When a family hurt by AIDS needed furniture, I donated my old couch and love seat. My wife and I wrapped presents for AIDS orphans at Christmas. I used each event, each national day of observance, as an excuse to write about AIDS. I received an award for my efforts from the South Carolina HIV/AIDS Council in Charleston in 2002.

In June 2003, I left South Carolina for Florida to work as an editor for the *St. Petersburg Times*. Journalists are nomads with short memories. We rarely look back. Each new job usually means new stories, new sources. But the story of AIDS in Clover refused to let me go. After two years of procrastination, I called Reverend Starr. Can I tell your story? I asked.

The initial encounter between reporter and speaker evolved into an education about HIV/AIDS in one of America's most vulnerable places. After countless telephone conversations, funerals, hospital and home visits, tears, and laughter, I came to understand and respect the fervor of those for whom fighting AIDS has become a crusade. Caring for people with AIDS is the kind of thankless work few are willing or equipped to do. Those dying of AIDS long for comfort, someone to hold their hands. No one wants to die alone.

This work is an attempt to break the silence, to provide a living memorial to the men and women in the shadows, those claimed by AIDS, those unfortunate enough to live in Clover, South Carolina, instead of more headline-grabbing places like Soweto, South Africa. This is an attempt to tell their story. In some instances names have been changed to protect the privacy of the living; in other cases I use the real names of those who died.

They didn't die of shame. No, the shame belongs to the living—the fool-hardy, obstinate survivors who refuse to acknowledge the real cause of their friends' and relatives' demises. AIDS or ignorance, silence or sex, the effect is the same. This is an attempt to invoke their memory and change the course of an ugly history.

THE FINAL CALL

The caller's voice sounded familiar, her urgency unmistakable.

"Can you come?" Reverend Patricia Starr asked, her words more summons than request. It was in the middle of the morning, but I immediately rose and walked out of my tiny office in the *Rock Hill Herald* newsroom. Five minutes later, I pulled my white Ford Taurus station wagon into the Piedmont Medical Center parking lot, walked through the automatic doors into the emergency room, and strode down the crowded hallway to the bank of elevators. As I rode up to the second floor, the gravity of the summons created a knot in my stomach and dryness in my mouth.

Reverend Starr met me at the door to the private room where her baby sister, Carolyn (pronounced *KERL-in*), lay gravely ill. As she had done for scores of others, Reverend Starr came daily to sit with her sister and comfort her. Her skills were sorely tested that day.

A week earlier, as dawn broke, Carolyn's young son had come running to Reverend Starr's house. His mother had passed out on the floor of her apartment and he couldn't wake her, he sobbed. Reverend Starr rose, pulled on a housecoat, and ran along the dirt path to Carolyn's apartment, where she found her sister frothing at the mouth and unresponsive, her eyes rolled back in her head.

After an ambulance rushed the unconscious Carolyn to the ER, she clung to life as doctors tried to stem the damage of what looked like a drug overdose. Their rescue efforts were frustrated because Carolyn was in no shape to say what illegal narcotic she'd injected. Tricia Ann, as friends called Reverend Starr, was furious. This wasn't Carolyn's first drug overdose. Her sister had spent much of the previous two decades on an endless narcotic binge. But now the stakes were much higher.

Carolyn had full-blown AIDS. She was tired. Did she have the strength to fight one more battle?

As a columnist for the local McClatchy newspaper, I had written about Carolyn's AIDS infection and her sister's mission to prevent others from suffering a similar fate. Tricia Ann invited me to Carolyn's bedside to say good-bye while there was still time. The hospital room was painted Carolina blue, just like the fabric covering the recliner where Tricia Ann sat next to her sister reading and answering questions. As Carolyn drifted between sleep and fitful awakening, Tricia Ann often struggled to determine which was which. Sometimes she'd begin reading aloud from her King James Bible, but Carolyn responded only with gibberish.

Familiar faces haunted the patient's bedside. Carolyn kept seeing her older brother Woody, who had died of complications from diabetes while she was in prison, and her mother, Annie Mae Pegram, whose death in 1979 triggered Carolyn's downward spiral into the world of illicit drugs and sex. In moments of enchanted lucidity, Carolyn chatted excitedly about a golden room. She repeatedly pointed to a man dressed in a purple robe who stood in the corner of her room. Her sister's hallucinations prompted Tricia Ann to begin rereading her old copy of *A Divine Revelation of Heaven*, Mary Baxter's bestselling book, which purportedly details scenes of a glorious afterlife. Ever curious, Tricia Ann wanted to see if Carolyn's ramblings matched Baxter's spectacular visions.

For almost a decade, Tricia Ann had kept watch as Carolyn's health ebbed and flowed, but her sister's afterlife visions had finally convinced Tricia Ann that Carolyn's long, dark journey might soon end. After all, as pastor of True Word of God Fire Baptized Holiness Church, Tricia Ann had ministered to countless people in their final days. Her life, it seemed, had always been consumed by concerns of first and last things. It was as if God had ordained her to watch her loved ones breathe their last, long before their time: her mother at age fifty, her brother at age thirty-five. It looked like fate had one final cruel twist: her baby sister at age thirty-five.

On that spring day, Carolyn lay in bed dressed in a plain nightgown. Despite the acne, it was obvious why the men in her hometown found Carolyn's high cheekbones and chocolate-brown face so tragically irresistible. The quietness that governed the room was soon interrupted by the firm, assured footsteps of Dr. Craig Charles. This wasn't the time for his usual early morning rounds. The doctor wore a somber expression, the look of a physician caring for a patient confronting grave odds. He was dressed in a knee-length white coat, white shirt and a tie, and khaki pants.

Dr. Charles had studied infectious diseases at Wake Forest University Baptist Medical Center in North Carolina before starting his medical practice in 1996. Five years later he moved to South Carolina, where he met Carolyn at the downtown Christopher Clinic, a center created by the Catawba Care Coalition to serve poor HIV and AIDS patients.

After dozens of visits, doctor and patient knew the routine and the language of AIDS—T cell counts and antiviral loads—that told the tale of AIDS destroying Carolyn's body. But that spring morning, as Dr. Charles sat at the foot of Carolyn's bed, his words were very deliberate. Tricia Ann sat at the other end of the bed, her sister's head cradled in her lap. Tricia Ann could see Carolyn's full round face, her eyes listless, bloodshot, a permanent optical tattoo from her years of abusing crack cocaine and heroin.

"This is the hardest thing for a doctor to do," he said. "Nothing is working. Her disease has progressed too far." As Dr. Charles spoke, Tricia Ann held her breath, afraid of what the physician was about to say. After all, it seemed as if her life, the life of her family, had been wrapped around a succession of grim-faced doctors' visits stretching back two generations. And for the previous six years, Tricia Ann had sat beside Carolyn listening to one doctor after the next give similarly dire predictions. Somehow time had proved them wrong. Carolyn was a fighter; she had beaten the odds before. Could she do it again?

But Dr. Charles' sober words swept away Tricia Ann's waning optimism like a sand castle before the frothy ocean surf. "I'm so sorry. I'm so sorry,"

Dr. Charles repeated. "As a doctor, I try not to get too emotionally involved with patients. But you guys have been there. It's hard."

His words hung in the air for what seemed like forever until Carolyn spoke up, her voice dry and hoarse, not much louder than a whisper. "What are you saying? I am going to die?" she asked, looking at her older sister, her eyes pleading as if for more time.

Tricia Ann said nothing. Both women stared at the white physician, who let Carolyn's words sit like untouched dinner. As if responding to her own question, Carolyn erupted in a torrent of tears and screams.

"I'm going to die. I'm going to die," she cried. Tricia Ann squeezed her sister's hands. A wave of helplessness engulfed her. This woman, who preached fire and brimstone for two hours on Sundays without notes or respite, could only grasp for words. For this moment, the power of speech failed her. Then the experienced pastor, who usually found the strength to buttress the suffering and dying in their most vulnerable moments, regained her voice, if not her composure.

"How much time do we have?" she asked tersely.

The physician took his time answering, as if bracing himself before he spilled more bad news. "Only God knows what time," Dr. Charles responded. "Given her condition, it won't be long."

The infection had spread throughout Carolyn's body. Her immune system was compromised and the antibiotics no longer worked. Her fever had spiked and her blood pressure had plummeted, he said.

Then Carolyn seemed to summon her last remaining dregs of resolve. "Tricia Ann, I want to go home," she said. Tricia Ann looked at the physician. "Is that possible?" she asked.

"I would let her go home under hospice supervision," Dr. Charles replied.

"Can you make that happen, right away?" she said, her response part request, part demand.

He then walked around Carolyn's hospital bed. He hugged her and then embraced Tricia Ann. For a moment, the enormity of the news seemed to cement the bond between physician and patient, healer and the sick. Dr. Charles looked Tricia Ann straight in the eye and held her gaze.

"The good part is that she has you," he said. "You know how to pray."

"I'm doing that," Tricia Ann said. At that moment, she felt overwhelmed by the physician's show of compassion, his sensitivity, his zest for his work. This doctor loves what he does, she thought to herself.

In her lifetime Tricia Ann had been in too many hospitals and known too many doctors to count. But rarely had she encountered a physician like Dr. Charles, who fought for his patients and invested so much in the outcome of their treatment. He didn't act as if he possessed the power of life and death, but he clearly was prepared to do everything he could to save a patient. And when he couldn't, he was the first to admit the limits of his skills and the constraints of modern medicine.

As Dr. Charles walked out of the hospital room, Tricia Ann felt the urge to follow him. She wanted to ask him questions he might have been reluctant to answer. She had mulled over every nuance of Dr. Charles's prognosis, but she felt he was holding something back, as if the news was too devastating for Carolyn's shredded psyche. Tricia Ann desperately needed to hear it, but sibling loyalty anchored her in place. At that moment, she belonged at Carolyn's bedside.

That was the way it was. Carolyn could always count on her big sister, even during the days when she ran the streets and sold Tricia Ann's clothes and food for money to buy drugs.

Before he left the room, Dr. Charles had promised to assign a nurse to bring a sedative to quiet Carolyn, who was crying hysterically. Seconds after the nurse injected her, Carolyn dozed off. As she slipped into a restful sleep, her breathing shallow but even, Tricia Ann tiptoed out of the room in search of Dr. Charles. When she found him, he accompanied her into one of those small hospital conference rooms where physicians and families are brought together by bad news.

"What are we looking at?" she asked.

"Her organs are shutting down; her kidney and liver are shot," he said. "Whatever they laced it with, it messed up her system. We've tried some of the strongest stuff we have, but it isn't working."

"Whoever did this really killed my baby sister," Tricia Ann thought out loud.

Dr. Charles didn't venture that far. "The disease didn't help," he said.

"They poisoned her," Tricia Ann insisted, anger and frustration welling up in her voice. Dr. Charles didn't agree or disagree. He had clearly moved on. The time for recrimination had long passed.

"If she has family, she needs to call them. Let her make her peace," he counseled. "We don't have much time." The physician's words held an air of finality. They sounded like words of benediction for a ritual Tricia Ann had experienced before. It seemed so familiar, yet so new. Over the previous five or six years, she had accompanied dozens of family members—mostly mothers and sisters—to the bedsides of young men and women dying of AIDS. She had tried to find the right words of comfort, to reassure the grieving that death, even the death of a loved one from AIDS, was all part of God's mysterious plan. She believed it, otherwise she would never have said it. But sitting in that same hospital, hearing the end was near, meant something very different when the woman in the bed was her baby sister.

To find solace, Tricia Ann tried to remember the easier conversations she had had in situations like this. There was the time she had accompanied a mother and sister to say good-bye to a thirty-seven-year-old man who was dying of AIDS. That day there wasn't much she could muster: "It's hard, the thought of burying your child. I could only imagine the hurt of hearing the doctors say they have done all they could," she told the woman weakly.

"My child is in God's hands," the mother replied.

Tricia Ann remembered the look on that mother's face as she got up and walked up and down the hospital hallway, as if pacing would make her son better. The woman had stopped and gazed out the window for a while, then started pacing again. By contrast, the dying man's sister, who had been his caregiver, was calm and controlled.

"When you know that you've done your best, it's a different feeling," Tricia Ann said. "You deal with it differently. Even though it hurts."

Part of her knew she had tried to do everything humanly possible to save her sister. Yet on that spring morning she found herself pacing the same hallways and looking out the same window as if searching for answers, the way that grieving mother had done.

She dug deep and came up empty. She wished she could have switched places with Carolyn and given her a chance to do it over again so her baby sister could get it right. She wanted her to experience the joy of knowing God, peace, and even happiness.

That was never Carolyn's fate. Starting from when she was a little girl, she only saw pain, anger, sickness, and betrayal. And long before she became a woman, she began to act in ways that guaranteed the cycle would continue.

Carolyn was too young to remember when her mother, Annie Mae Pegram, was healthy and strong enough to take the children to the grocery store on Saturday afternoons; she was not old enough to remember her father, Samuel Pegram, when he worked three jobs and found time to fuss over his children. The father she knew wasn't a father she could love.

By the time Carolyn was old enough to understand, Samuel Pegram was staying out all night and weekends, and Annie Mae Pegram was crippled by cancer, gout, and arthritis. Tricia Ann and her older siblings could treasure all their pleasant memories from happy times. Carolyn only saw misery. "I had my dad before he started going wild," Tricia Ann says. "She never remembered any of those things."

And so the little girl who grew up in misery lived every minute of her life pursuing happiness in all the wrong places. Nothing Tricia Ann said or did could stop Carolyn. A drug addiction can overpower a sister's love. Still, as Carolyn lay dying, Tricia Ann felt overwhelmed by a sense of failure, the feeling that she hadn't done enough to save her sister. She had failed Carolyn. She had failed her mother. "Momma wanted me to take care of her, and I let her down," Tricia Ann says.

The sense of powerlessness was palpable in Carolyn's hospital room. As she slept, I squeezed her hands and rose to leave, with Tricia Ann right on my heels. Without success, she tried to figure out the puzzled look on my face.

As I stepped inside the elevator, I saw a woman carrying what looked like a brand-new baby wrapped in pink, the color of the blanket and clothing suggesting she was taking home a daughter. I was immediately struck by the irony of what I had just witnessed, an unmistakable parallel of peril and promise: upstairs someone's baby girl hovered near death, downstairs a smiling mother headed homeward with a newborn baby girl all dressed in pink. Could that joyful mother even imagine what it would be like to watch her daughter suffer and die of AIDS?

Unfortunately, too many southern mothers had confronted that question. Since the first cases of AIDS appeared in 1981, the epidemic had spread way beyond the gay and intravenous drug–using population. Women like Carolyn had become the poster children for HIV/AIDS.

Even as Carolyn lay dying that spring, throughout the states of the Old Confederacy doctors, activists, social workers, public health administrators, and people with HIV/AIDS had begun serious discussions in a belated attempt to slow the spread of the disease in the South. Within a year, representatives from South Carolina, North Carolina, Alabama, Georgia, Florida, Louisiana, Mississippi, and Kentucky issued the *Southern States Manifesto* to warn about the government inaction, ignorance, illness, and illicit sex that made the South the front line in the domestic war against AIDS.

Eight of the top ten states in which the highest percentage of African Americans who have AIDS live are in the South, according to Centers for Disease Control and Prevention (CDC) statistics. In all of those states, the majority of people who have AIDS are African American. Six of the top ten states in which the highest percentages of women who have AIDS live are in the South, according to the CDC.

The South is home to the highest number of adults and adolescents living with and dying from AIDS in the United States. That trend seemed to have totally ambushed the experts. With AIDS seemingly under control and the threat to heterosexual America apparently abated, the world's focus shifted belatedly to the emerging pathological cyclone decimating the populations of sub-Saharan Africa—in Angola, Botswana, South Africa, and Kenya, thousands of children were being orphaned daily by the deadly virus.

Even as the world's gaze was turned elsewhere, AIDS spread in the states of the Old Confederacy like kudzu growing along a country road. Between

2001 and 2005, the number of AIDS deaths decreased throughout the rest of the United States but continued to rise in the South. From 2000 to 2003, new AIDS cases jumped by 36.5 percent in the half-dozen states that make up the Deep South—Alabama, Georgia, Louisiana, Mississippi, and North and South Carolina. Florida, Georgia, Louisiana, South Carolina, and Tennessee suffered rates of AIDS cases higher than the national average in 2005.

In 2005, half of all the funeral services conducted for people who died of AIDS were held in the South, in churches just like Starr's white clapboard True Word of God Fire Baptized Holiness Church. This death ritual had become all too familiar.

The South was home to 36 percent of the US population but 40 percent of AIDS cases, according to the CDC. The region's health care systems became increasingly overburdened as HIV/AIDS devastated vulnerable populations, especially poor black men and women. This region is dominated by small towns like Clover, "the town with love in the middle," that are rife with pervasive poverty, lack of adequate health services, poor infrastructure, high unemployment and underemployment, and too many people who can't afford health insurance. When you combine these factors with the severe lack of funding for HIV/AIDS care, it paints a dire picture for the South.

Even as other regions in America devised programs to stem the flow of AIDS, southerners remained bound by denial. A conspiracy of hypocrisy, shame, false morality, cowardice, and political opportunism conspired to keep AIDS, "God's curse on homosexuals," off the public policy list of priorities.

Nowhere was this story more evident than in Starr's home town, where the Clover Community Cemetery, the town's black burial ground, is littered with the headstones of dozens of black men and women who died too soon from AIDS. Carolyn would be spared the indignity of joining them. A grave was reserved for her in a family plot several miles away.

The CDC documented the first cases of what would later be called acquired immune deficiency syndrome in 1981. A year later, Dr. Robert Ball, a Charleston epidemiologist, treated a gay man with horrendous oral and genital herpes. He was South Carolina's first AIDS patient.

State health records show that the first case of HIV in York County, where Clover is located, was diagnosed in 1985. There were five more cases a year later. In 1987, six years after the arrival of AIDS on the national scene, fourteen York County residents were diagnosed with HIV.

No one knows for sure how or when AIDS reached Clover. Perhaps some felon returned from state prison with more than just the tattoos on his arms; maybe it was the woman who had moved up North and came back home when she fell ill but didn't get tested until long after she had shared her deadly secret with more than a few casual lovers; maybe it was one of the young men who had visited the gay clubs in Charlotte, the metropolis forty minutes to the north. No one knows for sure when it started, but they can remember when they first began to notice how formerly healthy men and women began to wither away in plain sight, their arms and legs growing skinny and frail, their dark skin pockmarked by lesions. And they remember the whispers, the rumors, but most of all the dying: Cliff, Sandy, Nita, Jackie, Carolyn, Tracy, Robbie, Girard, and all the others. It is impossible to say how many Clover residents died of AIDS, as South Carolina was notorious for lax infectious disease tracking in the early years. And some victims, dying of shame, left town or simply crossed the state line and died in neighboring Gaston County or in Charlotte, North Carolina.

By 2002 Carolyn had become the new face of AIDS. She was one of the thousands of young black women in small rural towns across America's Bible Belt dying of what many religious people believed was God's plague against gays. But she wasn't gay. She always loved older men and was driven throughout her short life by an insatiable hunger and a reckless search for the affection and affirmation denied her by a promiscuous, absentee father and a bedridden mother.

Carolyn craved the attention of the fifty-something-year-old men who stood on the street corners and leered at her as she strolled by. The two fit like hand in glove. Their lust for her and her craving for crack cocaine and heroin found mutual satisfaction in the dark alleys and shotgun houses of the Cloverdale neighborhood.

Even as America has dispatched billions to fight this disease overseas, our small rural communities remain vulnerable to the sinister threat of HIV/AIDS. The enemy isn't just the physical illness. It's ignorance; it's the guilt and shame-inducing silence that kills our young. It's time to end the silence and to provoke an eruption of empathy, compassion, and community action to alter the sad trajectory of AIDS in our small towns.

HIV/AIDS remains a significant public health and social justice crisis in the United States, and the South in particular is heavily burdened, warned the authors of the *Southern States Manifesto*. Poverty, poor education, and limited community resources conspire against people who live in the rural South. Through initiatives such as Southern REACH, the National AIDS Fund pledged to provide program grants to "strategically positioned" community-based organizations that have demonstrated the ability to reach priority populations with HIV prevention and care services or to lead policy and advocacy efforts.

"HIV/AIDS is more than a disease—it is a symptom of the larger problems of social inequalities and racial/ethnic health disparities," said Kandy Ferree, National AIDS Fund president and CEO, in a prepared statement. "Nowhere are such issues more prevalent in the US than in the South."

2

CAROLYN

Carolyn was a child of hope. She came into the world just when the dark clouds of racial oppression seemed ready to part and America looked like it was finally willing to live up to its promise of equality for America's twenty-one million black citizens.

She was born in 1964, considered to be one of the most transformative years for black folks in the century since Abraham Lincoln issued the Emancipation Proclamation. That year, President Lyndon B. Johnson launched one of the most ambitious socioeconomic initiatives ever and pushed through legislation designed to demolish the racially oppressive social and political order that had governed the states of the Old Confederacy since the last remaining Union soldiers had emptied their barracks, boarded trains, and headed north in the 1870s.

On January 8, 1964, even as Annie Mae Pegram waited for the first labor pains that would signal Carolyn's entrance into the world, President Johnson spoke to the nation in his State of the Union address. Johnson, who had ascended to the American presidency two months earlier following the assassination of John F. Kennedy, used the historic speech to declare a "war on poverty."

As Johnson's laconic Texan drawl traveled the airwaves, Annie Mae, nine months pregnant and swollen as a house, must have sat in her kitchen listening to the president's words over the radio. The stirrings of hope in her bosom must have grown stronger with each of President Johnson's pronouncements. He urged Congress to "let this session be known as the session that does more for civil rights than the last one hundred sessions combined . . . the session that declared all out war on human poverty and unemployment in these United States. The session that finally recognized all of the health needs of elder citizens . . . As the session which builds more homes, schools, libraries, and hospitals than any single session of Congress in the history of our republic." President Johnson spoke to bursts of applause.

Against all odds, Johnson tried to pry the Pegrams and millions of others from the stranglehold of poverty. He hoped to deploy a series of educational, health, nutritional, and community development initiatives to lift the chronically poor, one-fifth of the nation's population, from the generational grip of destitution.

Johnson acknowledged that he was swimming against the tide of recent history as he tried to nudge a reluctant nation away from its racially troubled past. Knowing the difficulty of the task, the big Texan invoked the name of the fallen President Kennedy.

"We have in 1964 a unique opportunity and obligation—to prove the success of our system; to disprove those cynics and critics at home and abroad who question our purpose and our competence," Johnson said. "If we can forge a greater sense of unity, then and only then can we take full satisfaction in the state of the union."

Perhaps Annie Mae listened to President Johnson's speech alone, or maybe she herded her children into the kitchen to listen with her. But listening to a recording of Johnson's speech almost fifty years later, it is easy to imagine the optimism that his words must have stirred in the hearts of Annie Mae, her neighbors, and millions of other black Americans.

"Our joint federal-local effort must pursue poverty, pursue it wherever it exists—in city slums and small towns, in sharecropper shacks or in migrant worker camps, on Indian reservations, among whites as well as Negroes, among the young as well as the aged, in the boom towns and in the depressed areas," Johnson said.

Annie Mae came from generations of sharecroppers. They picked cotton and tobacco and performed menial labor as they tried to eke out a living during those dark years after Reconstruction and the first half of the twentieth century. As many of her friends and neighbors boarded trains and buses and fled north to escape the cruel uncertainty of life under Jim Crow, Annie Mae stayed and prayed for liberation. But like her parents before her, Annie Mae despaired of finding release from the yoke that rested heavily on their shoulders. Her ancestors had heard presidents and politicians promise freedom and liberty, but they had only collected crumbs. She was not audacious enough to believe that change would come in her lifetime, but she hoped that it would arrive in time for her children and grandchildren.

The first stirrings of change were apparent even before President Johnson spoke his historic words. For more than a decade, black folks in the South had shown their unwillingness to wait for whites to hand them equality and justice. They were restive and ready. The news, in newspapers and on radios and televisions, was filled with reports of blacks across the South protesting, standing up for their civil rights, sending the message that they were tired of living as second-class citizens a hundred years after the Fifteenth Amendment granted them the full rights of citizenship.

While Annie Mae was willing to wait on the Lord for salvation, a younger generation of South Carolinians, mostly college students, was tired of waiting. These students took their cue from activists like John Lewis and leaders of the Student Nonviolent Coordinating Committee, who had brought civil unrest to Georgia, Mississippi, Alabama, and elsewhere in the Deep South. About twenty miles east of Clover, in the city of Rock Hill, nine students from Friendship Junior College were arrested in 1961 for demonstrating against segregated lunch counters. The group, dubbed the Friendship Nine, made national headlines after they decided to serve thirty days of hard labor in county jail rather than pay the $200 fine and be set free. President Johnson's speech must have sounded like a vindication of those young students' heroic actions.

"Unfortunately, too many Americans live on the outskirts of hope—some because of their poverty and some because of their color, and all too many because of both. Our task is to help replace despair with opportunity. This administration declares today, here and now, an unconditional war on poverty in America.

"Let me make one principle of this administration abundantly clear: All of these increased opportunities—in employment, in education, in housing, and in every field—must be open to Americans of every color. As far as the writ of federal law will run, we must abolish not some, but all, racial discrimination," Johnson intoned.

"For this is not merely an economic issue, or a social, political, or international issue. It is a moral issue. . . . All members of the public should have equal access to facilities open to the public. All members of the public should be equally eligible for federal benefits that are financed by the public. All members of the public should have an equal chance to vote for public officials and to send their children to good public schools and to contribute their talents to the public good."

Despite Johnson's lofty rhetoric, black folks had reason to be skeptical, to hold their expectations in check. A decade earlier, in 1954, the US Supreme Court had ruled in *Brown v. Board of Education* that separate but equal schools were unconstitutional. That decision was supposed to end the shameful social order that allowed white children to attend clean, well-kept schools while black children still attended classes in run-down, poorly heated buildings and read from outdated textbooks taught by teachers who were paid half as much as their similarly qualified white counterparts. But it didn't.

South Carolina legislators denounced the high court's desegregation ruling. Communities from the Atlantic to the Pacific sought ways to defy history and delay the inevitable. And Clover was no different. In 1964, Tricia Ann's older siblings still walked up the street to the all-black Roosevelt school. Few stayed past the sixth grade. Persistent inequality and the demands of everyday life demeaned their education. It wasn't worth waiting around for a high school diploma if the color of their skin disqualified them for all except menial jobs.

With President Johnson's words still ringing in her ears the morning after, Annie Mae buttoned her coat against the January chill as she prepared to drive ten miles east with her husband, Samuel, to Divine Saviour Hospital in York, the county seat.

Annie Mae wasn't perturbed about her upcoming trip to the hospital. She had been there eight times before. And each time she returned home with a bundle of joy—five dressed in blue, three dressed in pink: John, Mary Ann, Woody, Betty, Danny, William, Tricia Ann, and Spanky.

As Annie Mae readied herself, Tricia Ann stood anxiously nearby. The little girl was barely old enough to begin kindergarten, but she was already tired of the rough-and-tumble games her brothers played. She longed for someone to play dolls with, to play house like other girls do. So as Annie Mae struggled to button her coat over her protruding belly, Tricia Ann looked up eagerly at her, pleading for the gift she wanted more than anything else in the world. "Bring me back a baby sister from the hospital, Momma," Tricia Ann pleaded. "Bring me a baby sister."

Carolyn would be the fourth girl of the family, although only one, Tricia Ann, lived at home. Fate had intervened to take two of Annie Mae's other daughters. Her second baby, Mary Ann, lived for about a month before Annie Mae awoke to find the newborn cold and still. Doctors called it crib death. A few years later, Annie Mae gave birth to a second boy, Woody, and then another girl, Betty. But Betty suffered from chronic asthma and bronchitis. She wheezed and coughed her way through infancy. When Betty was four years old, her parents took her to live with Annie Mae's childless aunt, who could afford Betty's doctor bills.

After her mother left for the hospital, Tricia Ann didn't have to wait long to get her heart's desire. The next day, Friday, January 10, 1964, Annie Mae delivered a chubby, chocolate-brown baby girl. At the time, few black families in Clover could afford a telephone, so Tricia Ann had to await her father's return with the news that she had a baby sister.

Two days later, Annie Mae reappeared with a baby girl wrapped tightly in a pink blanket against the January cold. Tricia Ann could barely contain her excitement as she tried to kiss the newborn and touch her thick curly hair. Carolyn was blessed with a dark-skinned, round face accented by high cheekbones. She resembled a miniature version of her mother.

In January 1964, the march toward freedom and racial equality seemed unstoppable, like General Sherman's jaunt through the South a hundred years before. Two weeks after Annie Mae returned home with Carolyn, Congress ratified passage of the Twenty-Fourth Amendment to the US Constitution, prohibiting the use of poll taxes in national elections. Although the Fifteenth Amendment gave former slaves and their descendants the right to vote, Annie Mae and her ancestors rarely, if ever, tried to cast a ballot, because South Carolina and the states of the Old Confederacy had adopted poll taxes and literacy tests to stifle the political aspirations of successive generations of African Americans. The right to vote was tied to money and literacy. Annie Mae and her husband, Samuel Pegram, possessed very little of either. Their lives revolved around the daily struggle to feed, clothe, and shelter their seven children. Education and politics were luxuries neither could afford. It is unlikely that the two had ever cast a vote or served on a jury. When their neighbors ran afoul of the law and went on trial in the Civil War–era courthouse in York, Annie Mae and her husband were reduced to a place in the "colored" spectators' gallery, watching helplessly as the county's white citizens meted out their segregationist brand of justice.

She saw Ku Klux Klan crosses burning on her family's front yard when she was a girl. The Klan no longer rode by night in Clover, but, angered by the aggressive agitation of civil rights protesters, the resurgent Klan threatened to begin marching during the day. But Annie Mae never got into trouble. At an early age, she had perfected the two-step dance of survival and dignified subservience.

For generations, Jim Crow laws told black folks like Annie Mae where they could go and what they could do. And in case they forgot, WHITES ONLY and COLOREDS ONLY signs served as stark reminders. But despite white resistance, by the mid-1960s the old order was fraying at the edges. Facing the threat of black protests and boycotts in the state's largest cities in mid-1963, the segregation-era signs had largely disappeared from Main Street shops, restaurants, and theaters by the dawn of 1964. By fall of

'64, Congress passed and President Johnson signed the Civil Rights Act, which tried to do politically what judges had attempted but largely failed to accomplish from the bench a decade earlier. The legislation outlawed racial segregation in theaters, restaurants, hotels, public swimming pools, libraries, and public schools. Most important, it banned discrimination in hiring—an obstacle that had long frustrated the career aspirations of college-educated blacks, sapped their children's ambition, and stymied their socioeconomic mobility.

Congress could change laws, but legislation can never change the hearts of men. Even though the laws on the books spelled out equality, Annie Mae and her family faced the daily indignities of black life in a predominantly white small town. On the outside, Clover was an atypical southern town—no Civil War monument graced the town square, no plantation-era estates dominated the town's upscale neighborhoods. In southern historical terms, the community was relatively young. Unlike other southern towns that had been nurtured around cotton and tobacco plantations, Clover grew up around the railroad and later prospered from the arrival of textile mills. Since it was chartered in 1887, the town escaped the ravages of the Civil War and the political upheaval of Reconstruction in the years afterward. Its origins are rather utilitarian. The town was located at the site of a five-thousand-gallon water tank built to service the steam engines for the Chester and Lenoir Narrow Gauge Railroad. In the early 1920s and '30s, while other communities struggled through the Great Depression, Clover matured. Textile mills sprang up and flourished. Trains brought cotton from the fields in York and Chester counties and hauled away finished textiles to more lucrative markets in the Northeast and West.

The history of South Carolina for most of the twentieth century is the narrative of a black minority intimidated, exploited, and cheated by a racist, ruthless white majority. But it didn't start out that way. As late as 1920, the state possessed a disenfranchised black majority that was unable to flex its numerical muscles at the ballot box. But unlike many neighboring communities that boasted sizable, long-established black populations, Clover always had a smallish population of African Americans who learned to coexist with the descendants of the Scotch-Irish Presbyterian families who migrated south from Pennsylvania and Delaware along the Great Wagon Road and first settled in the area just south of Charlotte, North Carolina. Later they were followed by Germans, who established Lutheran churches in the communities south of the North Carolina state line. The Welsh Baptists came later. But all those migrants were ingrained with a religious and cultural conservatism that was passed down, undiluted, over the generations.

Several areas west of Clover experienced some of the most rabid anti-Reconstruction violence of the period. Spared the ravages of the Civil War and Reconstruction, Clover itself was never a hotbed of racialism. Still, the peace was maintained by a dance between a paternalistic white majority and an acquiescent, servile black minority, who represented about 20 percent of the town's population. Many of the black folks performed menial labor. But beginning in 1961, black men like Samuel Pegram were hired to work at the textile mills in town or across the state line in Gaston County, North Carolina.

When Annie Mae wasn't making babies, she dusted the pews, swept the floors, and burnished the stained glass at First Baptist Church of Clover, the all-white congregation that catered to the town's business and political elite. The church was founded in 1890 by a small group of Baptists who lived in a region dominated by Presbyterians. In the seventy-five years since its founding, the congregation had blossomed from upstart sectarian interloper to mill town establishment church. Each Sunday morning, judges, politicians, and bankers pulled up to the red brick building at 117 South Main Street knowing that every piece of furniture would be spotlessly clean thanks to Annie Mae's tireless efforts. She worked steadily, humming her favorite Negro spirituals and camp-meeting revival choruses. Most days she worked alone, reveling in her solitude. She scoured the pews and fished out the sealed envelopes stuffed with cash that had never reached the collection plate. Despite her poverty, she never considered keeping any of the money but gathered and deposited the cash at the church office.

Annie Mae was godly, loyal, and honest, just like the character in the 1959 movie *Imitation of Life*. She was a petite woman with a round brown face with dimpled cheeks that underlined her bright, sparkling eyes.

Annie Mae also helped make ends meet by ironing the clothes and cleaning the houses of Clover's affluent white families. It was an arrangement as traditional as the South itself, the classic relationship of black and white, servant and mistress, but one that Annie Mae didn't try to buck. Although she was not a learned woman, she understood the calculus of power in her small southern town. It was as if servitude were written into her genes; she worked hard for paltry pay and was always grateful for the relationships that could make her children's lives less difficult.

If Annie Mae's job at First Baptist Church of Clover helped provide for her family's material needs, her membership at Mount Olive Tabernacle Fire Baptized Holiness Church sustained their spiritual needs. Like many of her neighbors, she found solace in her religious faith after a lifetime of trouble and heartache. The summer she gave birth to her fourth son, William, Annie Mae met Jesus at a tent revival. Maybe it was the preacher's warning of perdition that changed the course of her life, or perhaps it was his promise of an afterlife of no more sorrows and no more tears, but Annie Mae believed. She was persuaded that God intervened in the affairs of men and that he would intervene to help her and her family. She taught her children not to fight but to trust God. And she lived by example.

So each Sunday morning and evening, each Wednesday and Friday night, you'd find Annie Mae and her children at the one-room wooden shack with the corrugated roof that sat across the street from the Pegram household. If, God forbid, the children were a minute late for Sunday morning service, they could hear the strains of tambourines, clapping hands, and joyous voices coming from the church.

Annie Mae loved to wear hats. She usually wore a prayer cap that sat on the top of her head, with her pressed hair hanging near her ears. Annie Mae didn't perm her hair. She pressed it with a hot iron comb that she heated on a charcoal stove. After she ran the hot comb through her jet-black hair, she used strips of brown paper to roll it.

EMMET O'NEAL LIBRARY
50 OAK STREET
MOUNTAIN BROOK, AL 35213

When the heat in the church grew oppressive with the singing and the clapping and the dancing, Annie Mae pulled out her Black's Funeral Home fan, the one with a picture of the proprietor, Sam Black, a big heavyset man, on the back. On communion Sundays, Annie Mae wore all white, with her prayer cap perched on her head. Hers was a covering, nothing like the Easter bonnets some women wore that would block the view of those sitting behind them. That wasn't Annie Mae's style. Church was about praising God and being blessed and refreshed to face the trials and troubles of the world come Monday morning.

Annie Mae made sure that every Sunday the whole brood was scrubbed clean, dressed in their best, shoes polished and shined, hair greased, ready to walk into morning worship. During prayer meetings, she brought a pillow for her knees. During song service, before Mother Mars preached her sermon, Annie Mae would stand to her feet whenever they announced her favorite hymn.

Go tell all my friends that my ship just came in, filled with the Holy
    Ghost, filled with the word divine
Don't you want to sail on a ship like mine?

Not far from where Annie Mae sat was her sister Jessie, who loved to sit in the Amen Corner to the right of the pulpit. She was just as fired up. When the spirit moved her, Jessie stepped out of her pew and danced down the aisle clapping and singing:

Let the Holy Ghost come flowing through
It will tell you just what to do;
If you let the Holy Ghost have his way,
It would keep you from going astray.

Jessie would throw her head back and yell, "Hallelujah, Hallelujah!" at the top of her voice.

Tricia Ann and her siblings watched the weekly spectacle with juvenile bemusement. Church was to be endured, not enjoyed. Annie Mae always sat in the second pew. As John and the older siblings reached their teen years,

EMMET O'NEAL LIBRARY
50 OAK STREET
MOUNTAIN BROOK, AL 35213

Annie Mae allowed them to sit to the rear of the church with their friends. But Tricia Ann, Spanky, and Carolyn, the youngest, most mischievous siblings, had to sit right next to their momma. Any wrong move was rewarded with a pinch—or worse, a stern look that would freeze their blood. When Annie Mae opened her soft eyes on them, it made them want to turn into a pillar of salt. It sent guilt racing through their very beings.

One Sunday, the family was singing and clapping in church as usual with Tricia Ann and Spanky standing next to their momma. As the congregation belted out the gospel anthem, Spanky seemed to be caught up in the spirit of the moment, singing at the top of his voice. Unfortunately, when his mother realized the young boy was singing the wrong song, she slapped him in the mouth and kept on singing without missing a beat. After the service, one curious church member who had seen Annie Mae slap Spanky came over to ask why she had punished her son.

"You didn't play in church," explains Tricia Ann. "You didn't get up during the preaching to go to the bathroom. You didn't move."

If Mount Olive Tabernacle Fire Baptized Holiness Church was a theater, the understated star was the preacher, Mother Mars. A petite widow, Mother Mars looked like a teacher, with a silver chain attached to her spectacles. Her husband had died of a stroke two years after they were married, and Mother Mars disregarded all suitors afterward. For forty-nine years she drove more than an hour from her home in Spartanburg to shepherd her small Clover congregation.

Mother Mars wasn't a showy preacher; she didn't have a throne on the dais. Before she stood to preach her sermon, she sat in the second pew, singing quietly with her eyes closed. Tricia Ann and the rest of the congregation knew when it was time for the sermon. As the ushers and deacons collected the offering, Mother Mars led the congregants as they sang:

I need you Lord, every hour I need thee
O bless me now my savior, I come to thee.

Then she rose and walked toward the pulpit. Her sermons always cut through Tricia Ann like a hot knife through butter. It felt like Annie Mae had told Mother Mars all of her family's secrets. The preacher seemed to be aware of Tricia Ann's mischief, because every Sunday morning it felt like Mother Mars preached about her.

One Friday, during an all-night prayer meeting, Mother Mars collapsed to the floor next to the podium, felled by a massive stroke. Men and women rushed to her side and desperately tried to revive her. Someone ran up the street to the nearest telephone to call an ambulance. By the time paramedics arrived, Mother Mars had regained consciousness. As she opened her eyes and surveyed the worried faces around her, the preacher made a stunning pronouncement.

"Y'all prayed me back," she said. "I was on the way to heaven. I saw my savior. Why didn't you let me go?"

That was Tricia Ann's first encounter with near death, heaven, and the afterlife. Years later as her mother, her brother, and then her sister Carolyn teetered toward the end, Tricia Ann remembered how Mother Mars had welcomed death without fear. That Friday night was the last time Mother Mars set foot in Mount Olive Tabernacle. She was admitted to a Spartanburg hospital and died soon afterward. Months later, the congregation renamed the church Mars Tabernacle Fire Baptized Holiness in their fallen pastor's memory.

Carolyn was much too young to know or appreciate the contentment in the Pegram household. Her mother, hardworking, patient, uncomplaining, and her father, Samuel, tall and thin as a reed, stood shoulder to shoulder to form a close-knit, proud, but poor family. During those early years, Samuel was the kind of daddy little southern girls adored. Unlike too many black men of his generation, he didn't abandon his children in poverty. He was a faithful provider. Each afternoon, plant supervisor E. J. Floyd drove down from Gastonia, North Carolina, in his station wagon to pick up Samuel and the other neighborhood men and drove them to work third shift at the Victor Dixie Village textile mill. Around midnight,

Annie Mae would hear the station wagon laboring as Floyd brought her husband back home. Although Samuel wasn't religious enough to accompany his wife and children to church on Sundays, in those days he didn't smoke, drink, gamble, or womanize. So after the vehicle pulled up in front of his house, he'd tiptoe inside so as not to wake the children and lay his six-foot-five frame next to his wife in the bed located in the living room. The children shared the two bedrooms—the older boys in one room, Tricia Ann, Spanky, and Carolyn in the other. On most mornings, before Tricia Ann walked to school, her father gave her a quarter to walk over to the old Neely's Store to buy him an Orange Crush soda and a pack of peanuts. He usually let her keep the change. On weekend nights, when he didn't work at the mill, Samuel was a bouncer at the Blue Light Café, a local speakeasy on Kings Mountain Street. He also worked at Black's Funeral Home. Tricia Ann loved to see her daddy looking gallant in his black undertaker suit as he drove the hearse or carried a casket to its resting place at the Clover Community Cemetery.

Carolyn was the baby of the brood, but her daddy treated Tricia Ann as if she were special. She'd sit on his lap, and he'd pat her and play with her. She was Daddy's little girl. Sometimes when Samuel headed over to the Blue Light Café or Black's Funeral Home, he'd take her by the hand and they'd stroll together, father and daughter, her little feet taking four steps to keep pace with each of his long, leggy strides.

If Tricia Ann idolized her father, she clung to her mother. The two sat together for hours in the kitchen as they peeled vegetables and cooked fatback and beans. Each Saturday after Annie Mae returned home from cleaning the church, she and Tricia Ann took the shopping cart and walked about half a mile to the white-owned Hagans grocery store.

Those weekly excursions should have been some of a young girl's fondest childhood memories. Instead, Tricia Ann remembers entering Hagans as a weekly ritual in humiliation.

Although the WHITES ONLY signs had been consigned to the attic, white folks still demanded the utmost respect from blacks. Disrespect could still spell bodily injury or death. Each Saturday evening, Tricia Ann was reminded of the status quo when she and her mother walked into Hagans and saw the gray-haired, rotund proprietor dressed in a blood-splattered white apron, a thick cigar gripped between his brown teeth. Tricia Ann despised the smell of tobacco smoke commingled with clotting blood; even more, she hated the way he spoke to Annie Mae and the other blacks without whose patronage the business might not have survived.

"What you want, nigger?" he'd asked brusquely. He coveted the business from black folks but was recalcitrant about giving them the respect they deserved. Inside the store, the Pegrams' subordinate station was reinforced each time the proprietor's granddaughter, a freckle-faced five- or six-year-old girl with a red ribbon in her blonde hair, looked Annie Mae in the face and spoke to the grown woman as if she were a child.

"What you want, gyul?" the little white girl asked, as if culturally bred to flaunt the social and political inequality between her and the older black woman.

"Yes, ma'am," Annie Mae responded to the little white girl's questions. "No, ma'am."

As Tricia Ann walked beside her mother, she fumed inside. She was furious about the way her mother seemed to grovel and bow down to someone white but so young. She wanted desperately to strike out and bash that little girl in her face for humiliating her mother. The seven-year-old black girl hated the white proprietor and all those white people in her little redneck town. "To them, we were just niggers," she recalls.

Tricia Ann remained sullenly silent as she and her mother picked up groceries, but the minute they stepped outside the store, she peppered her mother with angry questions.

"Why you answering 'yes ma'am' to someone who could be you own child?" Tricia Ann demanded, stopping just short of repeating the kind of disrespect the white girl had just displayed.

"You let God take care of it," Annie Mae said. "Just trust God." She responded to a higher power; her hope clearly lay in heaven. Each time Tricia Ann objected, her mother replied in the same long-suffering way that had helped her and her ancestors survive and endure four hundred years of racial subjugation.

One week, when money was so short that Annie Mae couldn't even afford to go grocery shopping, a Biggerstaff Furniture store salesman, whom they called the Blanket Man, pulled up in front of their house. They called him the Blanket Man because the salesman would pack the trunk of his car with blankets, bedspreads, and pillowcases to sell door-to-door to black families on credit. At the time, black customers weren't welcome to shop inside the Gastonia, North Carolina, store, but they would pay a little bit each week when the salesman made his rounds. That day the salesman showed up to collect his money for the bedspreads, but Annie Mae was broke. She told him so.

"I have to feed my family," she said. "If you want, I could get them off the bed and give them back to you." Of course, the salesman didn't want to take back the merchandise. Bed linens, even if spotlessly washed, were worthless once a black family had slept on them.

"Annie Mae, I will be back next week to get my money," the white salesman said before he climbed into his car and sped away.

She might have been devout in her religious faith, but Annie Mae didn't forget how to show righteous anger. One day during peach blossom season, she was sitting with Tricia Ann on the front porch while Samuel sat in his old station wagon flirting with some women from the neighborhood. Suddenly a bee landed on Tricia Ann's lip and stung her. The young girl was allergic to bee and ant stings, so her lip immediately began to swell. Her throat tightened, and she struggled to breathe. When Annie Mae realized what was happening, she called to her husband to drive their daughter to the nearest emergency room, which was about ten miles away. "Samuel!" she called.

"Samuel!" she repeated a second, third, and fourth time. When he didn't respond, Annie Mae stepped inside the house and picked up a .22 revolver and marched outside toward her husband. As she approached the vehicle, the women scattered like roaches from the exterminator. But Samuel was a little slow to react. By the time he saw his wife walking toward him with a ferocious gleam in her eyes and the pistol in her hand, he jumped out.

"Annie Mae, what are you doing with that gun?" His words were more a statement of disbelief than a question.

Annie Mae kept walking toward him and, without a word, pointed low toward her husband's long legs and pulled the trigger. The shot rang out. Samuel leapt in the air and howled in pain.

Annie Mae was a sure shot. The bullet had grazed her husband's toe. Seconds later, a curious neighbor who had heard the gunfire came to find out what the commotion was about. As soon as he saw the look on Annie Mae's face, he didn't need to ask. He offered to take Tricia Ann and her dad to the emergency room. When a nurse examined him, Samuel told her he had shot himself while cleaning the pistol.

That violent exchange was one of the rare moments of anger between Samuel and Annie Mae. At the time, it seemed to be a random, isolated incident totally at odds with the ebb and flow of life in the Pegram household. But like a starter's pistol, it signaled looming trouble, as family illness and a father's inattention combined to sow the seeds of marital discord and, eventually, a family's disintegration.

3

SOMEBODY ELSE IS WORSE OFF THAN YOU

One day in the winter of 1968, the winter after that long dismal summer, the same one when Dr. Martin Luther King Jr. was murdered in Memphis, Tennessee, the winter hard on the heels of the summer that Robert Kennedy was gunned down in a California hotel just when it seemed he was ready to win the Democratic presidential nomination and change the world again, that winter, as Annie Mae walked home on an icy cold day from her part-time job cleaning the floors and dusting the pews at First Baptist, she slipped on the ice and fell on the sidewalk in front of City Pharmacy on Main Street. In another place, another time, that fall could have opened the door to the Pegrams' financial fortune with a big legal settlement. But in 1968, a black woman who slipped on a treacherous municipal sidewalk in the Deep South must struggle to her feet and limp home. She must hope that the pain from the fall does not linger. In Annie Mae's case, that fall injured her back. She was never whole again.

After Annie Mae recovered enough to return to work, Tricia Ann and Woody accompanied their mom to clean the church on Saturdays. He buffed the floor; she dusted the pews. Their mother cleaned the kitchen, where she didn't have to climb. As she worked, she hummed her Negro spirituals and her camp-meeting songs. Her expression remained calm and pleasant, a ready smile leaping from her cheeks to her eyes as she serenely negotiated every obstacle. Even though her spirit was willing, her strength was failing.

Soon her gout and arthritis worsened and forced her hands and fingers to curl up in a clenched fist. And as her pain intensified, Annie Mae missed more time at work. For a while, the church kept faith in her. Annie Mae was the most honest custodian the congregation had ever employed. Any Sunday the offering plate was short, the treasurer could be sure that Miss Annie Mae would walk in Monday morning with the offering envelopes she'd found tucked into the back of the pews.

Eventually, though, they let her go. She couldn't keep up physically. The members gave her a small honorarium. Then she was left, without a pension, to fend for herself and her children. As her arthritis worsened, Annie Mae spent more time in bed. She couldn't even wash and iron clothes or babysit white children to earn a living. Then she was hit with an even direr prognosis.

One day, Tricia Ann and her brother William were arguing about whose turn it was to wash the dishes. As the siblings argued, Annie Mae walked into the bedroom and threatened to whip the pair if they didn't stop bickering. As she tried to grab William, he jumped across the bed, putting him beyond his mother's reach. In doing so, the teen broke a cardinal rule of the Pegram household.

"I'm going to get you," Annie Mae threatened. As she tried to stretch across the bed to punish him, Annie Mae stopped suddenly, clutched her chest, and slumped onto the bed, her usually serene countenance twisted and contorted in a painful grimace.

"Call John," she said weakly, as she continued to clutch her chest. Hours later, in the emergency room, physicians diagnosed Annie Mae with a mild heart attack. That scare, like a rooster crowing at dawn, signaled the first of more serious downturns in Annie Mae's health. Soon afterward she started bleeding, and her doctor admitted her to Gaston Memorial Hospital. She was gone for a week. The children, mostly oblivious to the adult conversation around them, paid no attention. But Tricia Ann eavesdropped on Annie Mae talking to her aunt. She had cancer. Even worse, it was ovarian cancer, the same illness that had felled her mother before she was fifty. Longevity seemed to be one gift that eluded her family. Later, while undergoing cobalt treatment, something went wrong. The radiation pierced her intestines. Annie Mae returned home with a colostomy bag.

At first Samuel tried to maintain intimate relations with his wife, but he found it impractical after a while. It didn't feel right. And, unfortunately, Samuel found it easy to find affection elsewhere, like many husbands with incapacitated wives have done.

As Annie Mae's health deteriorated, Tricia Ann became the de facto mother of the Pegram household. She was only nine or ten when she learned to make biscuits for the family. When Tricia Ann got home from school, she couldn't find a quiet place to complete her homework. She had grown-up responsibilities. While other children ran around and played, Tricia Ann cooked. Her siblings also had chores. The boys raked the yard, collected firewood, and fetched water. At four years of age, Carolyn was too young to do anything other than create a mess and get in the way.

Like most seriously ill parents who still had young children, Annie Mae tried to shield them from bad news, as if ignorance would protect them from her illness. Whenever one of her sons or daughters asked why she had to go to the hospital, Annie Mae always furnished the same response.

"Trust in God," she said. "Somebody is worse off than I am."

As Annie Mae was being treated for cancer, she suffered a stroke. Afterward she couldn't talk clearly because her mouth was twisted, a painful contortion of her once-beautiful smile.

Annie Mae's illness meant long hospital stays in Gastonia and Charlotte, North Carolina, and later, the Medical University of South Carolina in Charleston, 185 miles away. Illness also became an interloper in her marriage and her family's life. It shaped the children's days and nights and clouded their outlook. The children lived in fear of their mom's death. Twice, fearing the end, doctors called them to her bedside.

When the oncologists got tired of experimenting on her with new drugs, they sent her home to die. But Annie Mae was a fighter. She hung on for years—long enough to see Tricia Ann get married to her childhood boyfriend, Larry, and to see them start a family. But not long enough to see Carolyn grow into womanhood.

As his wife's health worsened, Samuel Pegram did what often comes naturally for a man of his age and situation. He stopped coming home from work. He stayed out late. On Friday evenings, he no longer brought his paycheck and placed it on the kitchen table. Some weekends, he didn't even set foot in the house at all. Soon the children heard the whispers and the rumors. As Samuel showered attention on Althea, a neighborhood teenager barely older than Tricia Ann, the children hoped and prayed their mother hadn't heard of their father's betrayal. Then one day when Tricia Ann was about thirteen or fourteen, she returned home from school to find Althea seated on the couch in the living room talking to Annie Mae. Blood rushed to Tricia Ann's face. Her only thought was that Althea had come to the house to hurt her defenseless mother.

"What is she doing here?" Tricia Ann demanded.

"Leave her be," Annie Mae replied calmly. "She needs help. She's coming to stay with us. She has nowhere to live. She's family."

Tricia Ann fumed that the two-timer and home wrecker was bold enough to come into their house. She felt like jumping on Althea and tearing her to pieces, but her mother's calm demeanor stayed her wrath. Powerless to hurt her mother's rival, Tricia Ann did the only thing she could think of. She turned and ran out the door and headed for her oldest brother John's house. John would know how to get rid of Althea even if Annie Mae objected.

"What is she doing here?" John asked his mother as he walked in the door.

"Don't mess with her. She's allowed to stay here," Annie Mae replied. "She has no other place to go."

"Have you lost your mind?" he asked. John was married and had his own family, but he and his younger siblings knew they had to respect Annie Mae, even though she was weak and disabled.

"This is my house. I'm going to let her stay here until she finds a place," Annie Mae replied.

To accommodate their new guest, Annie Mae moved Spanky, who shared a room with Tricia Ann and Carolyn, so Althea could sleep on his small bed. But Althea's stay in the Pegram household proved to be short. The very first night, Tricia Ann was awakened by the sound of her father sneaking into her bedroom crouched on all fours. The hinges creaked slightly as he turned the knob and opened the door just wide enough to crawl inside and climb into bed with Althea. Tricia Ann lay in silence, shocked by what she heard—the heavy breathing, the squeaking of the mattress springs—as the older man and the young girl came together in a brief tryst of betrayal. Tricia Ann's blood pounded in her head, and her heart beat so furiously it hurt her breasts. The heavy breathing and the groaning seemed to continue forever. As soon as it ended, she saw the silhouetted figure of her father crawl out of the room on his hands and knees, return to the living room, and climb back into bed with his sick wife. Within minutes, Tricia Ann could hear her mother whimpering in the dark, heartbroken by her husband's bold infidelity. As if it weren't bad enough that Annie Mae was being betrayed by her own body, now her husband was betraying her in the next room, under her own roof, with a girl she had taken in as a guest.

What she saw and heard that night robbed Tricia Ann of sleep. The teenager twisted and turned in bed and anxiously waited for the first signs of dawn seeping through the window. She could hardly wait to inflict vengeance on her philandering father and that ungrateful girl who spat in the face of Annie Mae's generosity. She wanted to dismember Althea; she wanted to grab a shotgun and murder her father. "I wanted to kill him," she says.

The next morning, as soon as she climbed out of bed, Tricia Ann told her siblings what had happened a few hours earlier. Her siblings hatched a plan to lynch Althea, but they needed their big brother John. So they dispatched Spanky, the youngest boy, to fetch him. Annie Mae must have known trouble was afoot, because once she saw the flurry of activity, she called her children each by name into the living room. As they filed in, she ordered them to sit. One by one they sulked in and sat, unable to disguise their anger.

"Save a seat for John," she said calmly.

Minutes later, as John burst through the door ready to exact revenge on his mother's tormentor, he came face-to-face with his mother, calm as ever.

"Take a seat," she said.

Annie Mae's tone whacked John's anger like a baseball bat against the knees, and he sank submissively onto the couch. With the accusers seated, Annie Mae summoned the accused, who hadn't yet emerged from the bedroom.

"Althea," she called. In the small wood-frame house, it would have been impossible for the young woman to be ignorant of the commotion she had caused. Annie Mae told Althea she couldn't guarantee her safety, given her children's anger.

"You have to leave," Annie Mae told her without raising her voice. "My children want to do you harm. And I can't blame them."

The Pegram children sat bunched together on the couch, frustration and anger etched on their faces. Tears ran down Tricia Ann's face while John sobbed as he struggled to control his temper. Even though he was a grown man, he could never defy his mother.

Shame and his children's disapproval failed to deter Samuel Pegram. In the absence of marital intimacy, he had lost all affection for his wife. Instead he found sexual fulfillment in his lithe, younger, more willing partner.

One day their predominantly black Cloverdale neighborhood came alive with the siren wail and flashing red lights of an ambulance. Word spread quickly that the paramedics had come to take Althea to the hospital. She was having a miscarriage. Samuel was at home, but when he heard what was going on he took off running. His long legs covered the distance to the idling ambulance in quick time. He didn't bother to ask the paramedics' permission. After he peeked inside and saw Althea on the stretcher, he climbed in beside her. The last his family saw of him that day was Samuel riding away in the ambulance accompanying Althea on the way to the emergency room.

Soon after that, Annie Mae was coming home from church in her wheelchair when she saw Samuel kissing Althea. Tricia Ann felt as if she could rip Althea apart limb by limb, but she knew her mother wouldn't let her. So she bided her time until she could avenge her mother's honor.

She didn't have to wait long. Several months later, Althea began taunting Annie Mae. She would stand in front of the Pegram house for hours cursing at the sick woman inside. She called her a cripple. She said Annie Mae couldn't take care of her man. Those taunting episodes and insults hurt Annie Mae to the core. It wasn't just that her husband was having an affair with a woman young enough to be his daughter, but here was Althea flaunting her affair in the cruelest way. Despite his wife's complaints, Samuel never intervened, and his young mistress saw his silence as license to continue. But Tricia Ann was prepared to take action. One day she returned home from school in time to overhear her mother's tormentor's taunts. She flew into a rage, rushed after Althea, and was about to beat her when a neighbor intervened.

Soon afterward Althea got pregnant again. Rumor had it that the baby was Samuel's, but Annie Mae didn't believe it. Her husband had a lousy prostate. He couldn't father any more babies. Of course, Samuel behaved as if the baby girl was his. It boosted his ego.

Once Samuel Pegram's heart left home, it was only a matter of time before his feet followed. Thursday, August 30, 1973, was a typically hot summer day in Clover. After a long vacation, the children were tanned and wiry from playing outside in the hot southern sun. The younger ones had begun to speak excitedly about returning to school after Labor Day. But their father contemplated a very different kind of beginning. Samuel Pegram loved and revered his old man. When his parents had divorced years earlier, Samuel, unlike his siblings, sided with his father and gained the enmity of his sisters and brothers. He adored his father and always sought his approval. Now his dad was dead. For Samuel, his father's passing was a curse and a boon. He felt exposed without his father's sage advice. But with his father out of the picture, he no longer felt constrained to continue his loveless, sexless marriage to Annie Mae. Despite his own failed marriage, Samuel's father had frowned on his son's philandering; he would have disapproved of Samuel abandoning his sick wife and children.

That Thursday Samuel buried his father. Tricia Ann and her siblings put on their Sunday best and drove with their father to the funeral. Their mother, sick and confined to a wheelchair, stayed home. After the service, Samuel accepted condolences from the other mourners and drove home in silence. He seemed preoccupied, as if building resolve for a decision he was about to make. When he reached the house, without greeting his wife, he walked into his bedroom and reached for his suitcase. Annie Mae, polite as ever, tried to make small talk. She asked her husband about the funeral and about relatives who attended the service.

"Everybody was fine," he replied.

Annie Mae suffered from cancer, stroke, gout, and arthritis, but she never stopped worrying about her husband. The way the children saw it, she always made him her top priority. "My mom always put my dad first no matter what he did or what he said," Tricia Ann says. "It was always about my daddy." Anne Mae loved Samuel until the day she died. Whenever any of her children uttered a disparaging remark about their father, Annie Mae rebuked them. "That's your daddy," she said. "If you don't love him you are shortening your days."

On that August afternoon, Annie Mae tried to do what she had done for years—break through her husband's sullen silence. She asked him how he was doing.

"Fine." Samuel answered each question without looking at his wife, without pausing. But Tricia Ann noticed a different tone in her father's voice. His words possessed a resignation, a coldness, as if he had made a decision he had chosen not to share with his family. Annie Mae sat near the door in her wheelchair and watched him pack his belongings into his suitcase. He was leaving for good.

"Whatever you do is fine," Annie Mae told him. "Whatever you do is fine."

Samuel packed his things in the trunk of the station wagon as Tricia Ann sat on the front porch watching him. As if trying to answer his daughter's unasked question, Samuel said, "Daddy is not happy. He got to go. Daddy loves you, baby, but Daddy's not happy. He's got to leave." Tricia

Ann's mind bulged with unanswered questions: How could he leave their mother in her crippled state? How would they put food on the table?

As soon as her husband drove away, Annie Mae turned her attention to her daughter. She knew Tricia Ann really loved her father despite his shortcomings, and she knew that her daughter was having a hard time coping with her mother's illness. Plus, it was her daughter's fourteenth birthday. She buried her grandfather and lost her dad on the same day, like attending two funerals instead of one. There was little to celebrate.

"Why don't you go somewhere and have some fun?" her mother urged.

"Momma, I don't want to go anywhere," the young girl resisted.

"I'll be all right," Annie Mae reassured her. "Go on now. I'll be all right. Somebody is worse off than me."

Years later the children would talk about the serenity on their mother's face as she watched her husband walk out the door, knowing he was never coming back. Tricia Ann fumed inside at her mother's acceptance of their new hardship. "Daddy left us. We were poor as dirt. We could be losing her. Who could be worse off?" she thought to herself.

As the years passed and she had a family of her own, as Carolyn's lifestyle spiraled out of control and the consequences became more severe, as Tricia Ann began to encounter people living and dying with HIV and AIDS, Tricia Ann always remembered her mother's words: "Somebody else is worse off than you."

Later that afternoon, Tricia Ann's oldest brother, John, came by. She told him her daddy had left. Samuel Pegram wasn't John's father, but the young man had treated him with the respect due to his mother's husband. Hearing of his stepfather's desertion, John cursed, but he was also glad Samuel had left. The older man's public womanizing was a constant source of embarrassment. "Good riddance," John said.

Annie Mae didn't want to dwell on her delinquent husband. She worried about Tricia Ann. "It's your sister's birthday," she told John. "Take her for a walk with you." John took his sister to the neighborhood café and offered her a sandwich and a drink. She declined his generosity, stood up, and, despite her mother's earlier admonition, headed for home. As she walked toward the house, Larry, one of her brother Woody's best friends, stepped out of one of the two nightclubs in their Cloverdale neighborhood and approached her.

"What are you doing out here, girl?" he asked, unaccustomed to see- ing Tricia Ann on the street. He offered to accompany her home; when she resisted, he persisted. "I'm going to walk you home. It's your birthday. I have a gift for you."

Without warning, he reached over and wrapped his arms around her and shoved his tongue into her mouth. The surprise kiss made her head spin and her stomach perform a somersault. Stunned, she pulled away and ran all the way home. When she stumbled inside, her mother was sitting up in bed.

"Larry kissed me!" Tricia Ann blurted out. "He put his tongue in my mouth."

She expected her mother to be upset, but instead Annie Mae laughed. It was the first time she had heard her mother laugh so heartily in a very long time. "You're such a gump," her mother said. "He likes you. Go get him."

The next day, Tricia Ann returned home from school to find Larry seated in the living room with her mother. He had come to ask Annie Mae for permission to date Tricia Ann. She couldn't believe how presumptuous he was. "I was furious," she says. "He didn't ask me. He asked my mother."

After that, Larry came over to the house regularly. Annie Mae never objected.

"That's the man you are going to marry," she teased. Tricia Ann thought Larry was rude and obnoxious, although he was one of her brothers' best friends. She felt his timing was wrong. She was in no mood to fall in love. All her emotions were centered on worrying about her mother and finding food to feed the family. A boyfriend was the last thing on her mind.

"I'm never going to marry that man," she protested. "Never."

No one listened to her.

4

I CRIED FOR YOU

Without Samuel's paycheck the Pegram family struggled harder than ever to keep hunger at bay. John, the eldest son, had his own family to feed, but he helped his mother with the bills; Woody, never a smart kid after an early bout of scarlet fever, dropped out of school and went to work at Edmond's turkey farm. His job came with more than just a paycheck. Employees were allowed to take home turkey parts damaged during slaughter. That meant the Pegrams had turkey to eat with their collard greens, green beans, and macaroni and cheese for Sunday dinner.

Annie Mae signed up for welfare. Once a month the family received food stamps and a check in the mail: $128 to feed a family of six. John would come to pick up the check and cash it. When Tricia Ann and her brothers took food stamps to Community Cash supermarket, they had to endure the snickers and taunts of white customers behind them in the grocery store checkout line, just like the insults and disrespect they'd received at Hagans grocery store years earlier.

Food stamps didn't go very far, but they paid for lots of beans: pinto beans on Monday, navy beans on Tuesday, black-eyed peas on Wednesday, snap beans or lima beans on Thursday. Friday's menu was a baloney sandwich.

When the beans and the salvaged turkey parts ran out, the Pegrams ate fatback and fried bread—white flour mixed with water and deep-fried in cooking oil. The fatback came from generous neighbors who slaughtered hogs.

Food stamps, however, weren't accepted currency at the woodpile. When the weather turned cold, the Pegrams couldn't afford to buy firewood, so the siblings trekked to the nearest textile factory and picked through the boxes of used cones, which served as fuel for the wood-burning stove in the living room and the potbellied stove in the kitchen.

Annie Mae surveyed the activity from her bed in the living room, unable to do much more than offer words of encouragement. And as her illness worsened, she was able to do less and less for herself. So in the mornings before Tricia Ann walked to school, she bathed her mother and made her breakfast. She prepared food for her to eat during the day and placed it on a tray where Annie Mae could reach it from her bed or wheelchair.

But even as she went to school and sat in the classroom, Tricia Ann thought only of her mother; she worried about Annie Mae being home alone, unable to walk to the bathroom. Annie Mae didn't want her daughter to quit school, so each morning she coaxed her out of the house to venture in search of a high school education. Sometimes Tricia Ann stepped out the door, walked down the street and around the neighborhood, then returned before noon. She told her mother that the teacher sent her home. Truth was, she couldn't concentrate on arithmetic and social studies while her mother had no one to care for her.

One hot spring day when she was not yet fifteen, Tricia Ann sat in the back row of her tenth grade classroom sobbing. Tears ran down her face and smudged the pages of her exercise book. Her teacher noticed, took the teenager by the hand, and led her into the hallway.

"Go home," she told Tricia Ann. It was all the excuse the young girl needed. She never set foot in that classroom again. "I did what I thought was best," she says. "I had to take care of my momma." Tricia Ann never regretted dropping out, only not returning to finish, but there was no shame in not having a high school diploma. Few people in her Cloverdale neighborhood had one.

Carolyn was too young to remember or appreciate a robust and healthy mother. She was four when Annie Mae fell on the sidewalk and injured her back. By the time Carolyn was ready to enroll in kindergarten, her mother couldn't accompany her on the first day of school. Tricia Ann held her baby sister's hand as the two walked to Roosevelt Elementary that September.

Although she was raised in a house full of children, Carolyn, the baby of the family, was left to fend for herself emotionally. She possessed none of the tools a young girl needed to cope that are typically provided by healthy and available parents. Unlike her older siblings, she had no reservoir of fond memories of a loving, nurturing mother and father to draw on. By the time she was old enough to acknowledge that nurturing, her father had long turned his attentions elsewhere. The August afternoon Samuel Pegram packed his belongings into his station wagon and left home, Carolyn was nine. She knew her mother only as the sickly woman who couldn't attend parent-teacher meetings or school concerts or even take her to the grocery store on Saturday afternoons the way Annie Mae had done with Tricia Ann years before.

As she grew, Carolyn was short and stout, her body full beyond her years. An old photograph Tricia Ann found around the house showed a pretty, dark-skinned girl. Dimples just like her mother's adorned her face. When she smiled, those dimples deepened like valleys, filling her face and her eyes with an allure men would find irresistible. She always had pretty hair, a magnet for the fawning hands of John and her other brothers. They loved to spoil her. She was their little girl. They bought her anything she liked. They went the extra mile for Carolyn for Christmas and her birthday, when it arrived two weeks after the holidays.

Tricia Ann and Woody played Santa Claus; they saved their nickels, dimes, and quarters to buy Christmas presents and hide them in the attic. One holiday season, they bought a white rocking chair. Woody bought Carolyn a baby doll with money he saved from his job at the turkey farm. Carolyn and Spanky were the babies, and their older siblings insisted on buying them presents in addition to the ones they got every year from the Clover Police Department toy drive.

Although her siblings did all they could to cheer her up, at some point, no matter what they did for her, Carolyn wasn't satisfied. She wasn't happy. "Why did Momma have to be sick all the time?" she asked. "She's never been there for me, no way."

Soon Carolyn wasn't a little girl anymore. Without able-bodied parents to instill discipline and rein her in, she rebelled early and often. As a fifth-grader, she played hooky and repeatedly threatened to quit school. Her pre-pubescent mind could not envision any need for an education. In elementary school she was cheeky, but she left most of the fighting to Tricia Ann. As she grew and entered middle school, her cheeky behavior turned vicious. If someone looked at Carolyn in a funny way, it was enough to start a fight.

She was defiant at school and at home. Under Annie Mae's rules, Carolyn was supposed to be in the house when the streetlights flicked on at sundown. But many evenings, long after the sun had disappeared behind Kings Mountain and the streetlights glowed gold and luminous, Carolyn still roamed the neighborhood. Usually Annie Mae deputized John to fetch his baby sister. He knew where to find her because Carolyn took to hanging around at one particular house, where women and older men sat talking, smoking, and drinking under an oak tree in the back yard. Some nights when her siblings thought she was safely tucked in bed, Carolyn slipped out through a rear window to run the streets. Each time, Annie Mae would summon John to bring her home. Too often he found her, a little girl acting more grown than her age, in the company of older men charmed by her high cheekbones, her dimpled smile, and her feisty spirit. Regardless of how many times they beat Carolyn or warned her about the company she kept, it only seemed to fuel her defiance.

Despite Carolyn's chronic rebellion, sympathetic adults never stopped trying to steer her in the right direction. A Clover Middle School teacher, Miss Brown, was one of those adults who took a special interest in Carolyn. She tried to encourage and counsel her, but to no avail. The young girl had set her eyes firmly on the streets.

One day, Miss Brown brought Carolyn home from school. She wanted to talk to Annie Mae. The teacher was aware of the situation in the Pegram household and knew Carolyn was having a hard time coping with her mother's illness. Carolyn felt abandoned and unloved. And she was in no mood to listen. She stormed off into her room and slammed the door shut behind her. Miss Brown told Annie Mae that Carolyn was angry because her mother was always sick. The teacher said she understood but warned Annie Mae that the school principal was losing patience. He'd expel Carolyn if her behavior didn't improve. Carolyn overheard the conversation from inside her room and chimed in. "They can kick me out if they want," she shouted. "I don't want to go no way."

Tricia Ann jumped to her feet and went after her. She wanted to grab her younger sister and slap her in the face for disrespecting her mother. "You can't talk to Momma like that," Tricia Ann shouted. But Carolyn only laughed at her older sister.

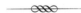

After Larry received Annie Mae's blessing to date her daughter, he courted Tricia Ann daily. Gradually he won her over; her resistance soon turned to romance. She grew to love him. As her mother slept, they smooched in Tricia Ann's small bedroom. Those delicious moments in the dark helped her forget the pain of her mother's illness. Larry was patient. Tall and handsome, he was accustomed to his girlfriends giving in to his desires within the first or second week. But not Tricia Ann. She was scared. Her resistance wasn't a badge of honor but a sign of insecurity. She had heard that boys loved girls with sexual experience. She was afraid to go all the way, and Larry grew to respect her for that. She was a fifteen-year-old virgin. That made her special. She wasn't like the other girls. Larry waited for eight months—a personal record for him. Eventually, though, as it usually does with young love, the couple's furtive kisses in the dark gave way to the irresistible impulse of sexual intercourse. At first they tried their best to hide their trysts from Annie Mae. Wise and circumspect, she already knew, but she never let on that she did.

After Tricia Ann lost her virginity, the naive country girl never considered that her excursions with Larry down the pathway of love would bear consequences. Even when her period didn't arrive on schedule, then was one, two, three weeks late, it never occurred to Tricia Ann that anything was amiss. But as her midsection began to harden and her breasts grew, Tricia Ann became aware of her condition. She was pregnant. She panicked. Larry offered to take her to an abortion clinic across the state line in North Carolina, but she refused. She wanted her baby.

But after all they'd been through together, how would she break the news to her mother? After all the admonitions and Bible scriptures about the wages of sin, she had behaved like the other girls down the street. She feared her momma's righteous wrath, but she feared the consequence of taking her unborn child's life even more.

Every day, she waited for the right time to break the news to Annie Mae. One day, while she was sorting through boxes of clothes that were too small for her and her siblings, she popped the question to her mother, who sat nearby in her wheelchair.

"Momma, what if I got pregnant?" Tricia Ann asked. Annie Mae remained silent for a moment as if she hadn't heard the question.

"Momma, what if I got pregnant?" she repeated the question.

"Nothing you can do about that," her mother replied. The response surprised her daughter speechless and liberated her to tell the simple truth.

"Momma, I'm pregnant," she said in a near whisper, as if uttered by someone else. Tricia Ann braced for an explosion that didn't come. Annie Mae never failed to surprise her daughter. She must have known the truth even before Tricia Ann opened her mouth because her short, calm response could only have come after long contemplation.

"You are grown up now," Annie Mae replied quietly. "Fun days are over."

Tricia Ann's life seemed to be moving at lightning speed. She had dropped out of school at fourteen; she became a mother at sixteen. Annie Mae was delighted when Larry asked for permission to marry Tricia Ann. But she didn't want him to marry her daughter out of a sense of obligation because she was pregnant. Tricia Ann needed someone to care for her after her mother was gone. Larry was a good man, her mother said.

"He won't love you the way you love him," her mother cautioned. "But that's OK."

The couple's first son, Santo, was born in August 1975. They married that October. Larry moved in with Annie Mae, Tricia Ann, and the rest of the family—Carolyn, Spanky, Woody, William, and Danny, and the brand-new baby boy. Annie Mae loved her grandbaby Santo. He slept in the bed next to her. She fed him and changed him. But the small house on Watson Street was too crowded for a married couple, mother-in-law, siblings, and a young child. The newlyweds needed a home of their own.

Several months later, when Larry's sister was visiting from Philadelphia, she took him and Tricia Ann to Gastonia to look for a place to live. They found a three-room house. She paid the deposit and their first month's rent. Tricia Ann and Larry bought their first piece of furniture, a couch, from Biggerstaff Furniture, the same store that used to send the door-to-door salesman to sell them linens in Clover.

The move to Gastonia complicated rather than simplified Tricia Ann's life. Now she was mistress of not one but two households. Each morning her husband drove Tricia Ann to Clover, where she spent the day taking care of Annie Mae and Santo. Larry returned in the evening, and they drove home to Gastonia. Soon they grew tired of that arrangement and found a place for Annie Mae and the kids to live near them in Gastonia. With Annie Mae settled down the street, Tricia Ann sometimes left her baby boy with Annie Mae overnight. They'd lay him beside his grand-mother with a bottle of milk and a few diapers. She could feed and change him without having to get out of bed. Her baby grandson was better company than Carolyn.

One Friday evening when Tricia Ann and Larry arrived at her mother's, Annie Mae was uncharacteristically irritable. She complained that Carolyn, in her haste to return to whatever she was doing, had reinserted her catheter tube incorrectly. Annie Mae wasn't sure what was wrong, but she didn't feel right.

When Tricia Ann lifted the bedspread, she saw her mother lying in a pool of blood that had soaked through the mattress. The sight of all that blood made her furious, and Tricia Ann stormed to Carolyn's room. The door was shut but not locked. Clearly Carolyn did not expect any interruption. When Tricia Ann barged into the dimly lit room, her baby sister lay in bed stark naked, cavorting with a grown man. Tricia Ann screamed at her and then at her lover. "Get out. Get out!" she yelled at him. "I should report you to the police for having sex with a child."

As the man scrambled for his clothes, he protested that Carolyn had lied to him about her age. In all the commotion, Carolyn didn't even budge. She just lay there naked, defiantly staring at Tricia Ann, who then reached out and grabbed her. Carolyn fought back like a hellcat, but her juvenile petulance was no match for her older sister's rage. Tricia Ann grabbed her by the hair, pulled her outside, and proceeded to administer a whipping that could be heard above the usual Friday night raucousness of the neighborhood.

Despite all the songs and all the fiery sermons she heard at church, for a long time Tricia Ann didn't believe in God the way Annie Mae did. But she never gave up on God. As she grew older and her first baby boy arrived, she continued to regularly attend church out of habit. Even after she was married in 1975 and moved to Gastonia, North Carolina, Tricia Ann still found time to go to church. But that's all she did.

Two years later, though, all the church attendance started to catch up with her and Larry. One Friday night in 1977 as most of the Clover townsfolk gathered in the high school gym for the heated York-Clover basketball game, Larry and Tricia Ann visited the home of a local pastor for counseling. Larry needed to talk. Tricia Ann went along for support. She remembers how that night Larry knelt at the couch in the living room and asked God for forgiveness. When he stood up he seemed relieved, as if the weight of a thousand transgressions had been lifted from his shoulders. He got saved. As they stood in the house, the presence of God hung heavy in the air. Then the preacher looked at Tricia Ann. "Do you want to get saved?" he asked.

"No. I'm not ready," she replied. A week later, Tricia Ann attended church to see the Carter Sisters anniversary concert. As she sat at the back of the room, the songs spoke to her heart. She felt the irresistible tug of her mother's faith drawing her forward to the altar. She didn't go up that night, but her resistance was beginning to crumble. The following Sunday as Tricia Ann again sat in church, it was as if the female preacher had been watching her all week. Her words stung.

"God got a hold of me," she said. The minute Tricia "got saved," all those conversations with Annie Mae began to make sense. She understood her mother's hope in spite of hard times. And over the next two years, Tricia Ann became aware of another calling. It said: preach. "I would laugh," she said. "I couldn't be no preacher."

After all, she was a high school dropout. Her formal education had barely progressed past the ninth grade. She didn't have the style and the poise to stand in front of a congregation and preach. Still, the voice persisted, though she tried to ignore it.

One day she was driving to York, South Carolina, when the words of Luke 4:18 popped into her head: "The spirit of the Lord is upon me to preach the gospel." Tricia Ann knew she couldn't ignore the call forever. But she had responsibilities; she had two young sons and an ailing mother to care for. Days later, Tricia Ann left her sons with her mother and drove home to pray. As she tells the story, while she was in her bedroom praying she fell into a trance. She saw herself bowing before the throne of God, then hollering that same scripture at the top of her voice.

"The spirit of the Lord is upon me to preach the gospel!"

When she came to, she was yelling so loudly that several construction workers who were working next door came and knocked on the window and asked if she was all right. "From that day I accepted my calling," she said. "The hardest thing was telling Momma that God had called me to preach."

When she finally told Annie Mae, her mother's response was puzzling. "I know God is going to call Larry" was all Annie Mae said, as if God had told her something he hadn't told her daughter.

Tricia Ann's pastor wasn't surprised to hear the news that one of her members felt called to preach. "She said, 'I knew.' I'm like, Why didn't anyone tell me?"

That was in 1977. In their church, being called to preach didn't require a seminary education. Right away, Tricia Ann began informal tutoring with her pastor. Soon afterward she was ready for her first sermon. That Sunday morning kinfolk from both sides of her family filled several pews of York Mount Zion to hear Tricia Ann preach on John 11:44 about Lazarus, the man Jesus brought back to life. Her message: Loose him and let him go. "I remember saying we can get our lives so tied up, but when Jesus calls, we can come out hopping or be still bound," she said. "He said loose him and let him go and the grave cloths fell off. I'll never forget my first message."

But letting go of her insecurities was hard. She didn't doubt her calling, just her ability to fulfill it. Thankfully, Larry was supportive. Whenever she preached, he would sit at a particular spot in the congregation, his eyes fastened on her. She would look in his direction, and he would give her a thumbs-up if she was doing a good job or a signal to calm down if she was speaking too fast. "I wouldn't be nervous if I focused on him," she said.

In 1979, two years after she first stood behind the pulpit, Tricia Ann obtained her preacher's license. In time, she began holding services in her home and eventually became the pastor of a church of her own.

Carolyn was unreliable. She couldn't be counted on to save her invalid mother in case of an emergency. Annie Mae knew that, and so did her other children. So, with Annie Mae's health worsening, Tricia Ann and Larry could think of only one solution. She would live with them.

The last years of Annie Mae's life were marked by intervals of respite and hospitals. Doctors would summon her children to her bedside for what they thought was a final good-bye, but time and again Annie Mae rallied. Her search for a cure took her to Gaston Memorial, to Carolinas Medical in Charlotte, and eventually to the sprawling Medical University of South Carolina campus in Charleston, where Annie Mae spent a whole year in the cancer ward undergoing the latest experimental treatments. Physicians knew that the drugs would never cure Annie Mae's ovarian cancer; the patient knew that too, but she willingly allowed herself to be a guinea pig for the betterment of science and future generations.

During that long hospitalization, Annie Mae's older children tried to stick together. Spanky and Carolyn, the only two minors, were farmed out to relatives. Spanky flourished. His aunts loved him. They treated him like a prince. Carolyn shuttled between John and her aunts as one after another relative tired of her promiscuous behavior. She learned fast how to use her body as currency to get whatever she wanted. Many nights she painted her eyes with shadow, brushed blush over her round cheekbones, emblazoned her lips with red lipstick, and sashayed down to the street corner, where grown men sought to reward themselves after a hard day of work.

When Annie Mae left Clover, her sons finally felt the freedom to live as they wished, too, knowing that their mother would have deplored their choices if she had been there to see them. William, her third son, chose hustling as his path to escape the stifling poverty he had known his entire life; he longed to eat steak, not the gravy and fried bread of his boyhood. He loved to gamble, but he was as lucky as a man with an expired lottery ticket. Eventually he turned his entrepreneurial talents to the illicit narcotics trade. He stalked the streets, wheeling and dealing cocaine or heroin, whatever the neighborhood junkies craved. But drug dealing was just another kind of gamble, one with higher stakes.

One Saturday night in May 1979, even as the rest of the family worried about Annie Mae's health, William was partner to a near-fatal transaction. A rival drug dealer shot William with a hollow-point, cop-killer bullet that severed an artery in his leg. William almost bled to death. While Annie Mae lay comatose at Carolinas Medical in Charlotte, thirty miles to the southwest in Gastonia, North Carolina, surgeons frantically fought to save her son's life. Tricia Ann and Larry received the news about William's injury as they sat in church Sunday morning. As they prepared to visit their brother's bedside, they received a summons from Charlotte. Doctors said Annie Mae's condition had worsened dramatically. After more than ten years, the end was near. John and his brother Danny drove from Clover to Gastonia to see William while Tricia Ann and her husband headed to her mother's bedside. Annie Mae would never hear about William's close call.

As Tricia Ann walked into the hospital room, Annie Mae opened her eyes briefly for the first time in a week. She hadn't said a word in twice as long. Annie Mae just turned her head to survey the room. Tricia Ann stood to the left of the bed; Uncle Zeb, Annie Mae's brother-in-law, stood at the foot. When the nurse came in to change her colostomy bag, Annie Mae opened her eyes, looked at Zeb and Tricia Ann, and smiled weakly.

"She's coming out of it," Tricia Ann optimistically said to the nurse. Annie Mae looked at them for a long, final time.

"Do you see me?" Tricia Ann asked repeatedly. Annie Mae looked at her visitors with her trademark serene smile. Then she turned her head and looked toward the far corner; as she did, her face lit up as if the sun had risen in the room and its glory reflected undimmed from her forehead, cheeks, and eyes. Annie Mae's gaze seemed fixed on a far-off destination. By the time the nurse had alerted the doctor and he arrived in the room, Annie Mae had closed her eyes again. Her breathing slowed. She lay still. She was gone. It was quick.

"Don't leave me, Momma, don't leave me," Tricia Ann screamed in vain. Annie Mae had hung on way past any of the most optimistic prognoses of the legions of oncologists who saw her during the previous decade. She had endured every test, every experimental cancer drug, and now she was free. It was Memorial Day, May 28, 1979.

Tricia Ann loved her momma dearly. She thought that no other loss could compare. She could never have imagined that the scene in the Charlotte hospital would be played out again and again, as a new illness, ten times more vicious than her mother's cancer, would stalk her siblings and her friends in Cloverdale.

5

BAD BLOOD

A nnie Mae Pegram's death in 1979 liberated her children from the constraints of her pious eyes. For the first time, they could pursue their
dreams and indulge their passions knowing she would never again call them
to account for their actions.

For most of them, this meant that they could enjoy as many sexual
partners as they desired. Their only worry was the inconvenience of catching syphilis, gonorrhea, or one of the other sexually transmitted diseases
that frequently circulated through poor rural neighborhoods like theirs in
Clover.

The scourge of STDs had not gone unnoticed. On Wednesday, June
13, 1979, two weeks after Annie Mae died, fifteen expert groups convened
at the Centers for Disease Control offices in Atlanta for the Conference
on Preventing Disease/Promoting Health Objectives for the Nation: Sexually Transmissible Diseases. Their mandate over the next forty-eight hours
was to draft working papers listing disease prevention and health objectives for the upcoming decade. Among the working groups was a team of
physicians, researchers, educators, community activists, and city, state, and
federal public health officials brought together to focus on the fight against
sexually transmitted diseases. At the table sat researchers and scholars from
Purdue University in Indiana, the University of Wisconsin, and the University of Washington; there were also state and municipal public health
officials, including Douglas Morgan, who represented his hometown of
Newark, New Jersey. Although Morgan didn't know it at the time, his work

on sexually transmitted diseases was preparing him for confronting AIDS, which would become his life's work.

Morgan earned his master's degree in public health at New York University under the tutelage of Dr. Lowell Bellin, the New York City health czar during the financially troubled mid-1970s. They spent most of their class sessions debating the city's crippling fiscal plight. Soon after the Atlanta conference, Morgan left to work at the Robert Johnson Foundation and later for the state of New Jersey before returning in the mid-1980s to direct his hometown's fight against the new threat of HIV and AIDS. Three decades later, Morgan was in Washington working for Health Resources Services Administration on Ryan White CARE Act initiatives.

Other than the Atlanta-based CDC officials, the South, a region persistently plagued with cyclical epidemics of syphilis and gonorrhea, lacked substantial representation at the table. Before they began their two days of "spirited and controversial" deliberations, Morgan and his fellow participants were handed a thirty-page dossier on the fight against STDs, especially syphilis, gonorrhea, and chlamydia. Those background briefing papers would have detailed America's century-long effort to stem the spread of syphilis among the general populace and especially among African Americans in the South.

Caused by *Treponema pallidum*, syphilis has been dubbed the "great imitator" because many of its symptoms mimic those of other diseases. Catching syphilis is simple: have unprotected vaginal, oral, or anal sex with a partner who has the moist, early lesions of primary or second-stage syphilis. What conference attendees would not have known then was that syphilis, an ulcerative genital disease, would efficiently facilitate the transmission of the worst STD imaginable—the human immunodeficiency virus (HIV)—creating an unfettered expressway to AIDS. In years to come, when understanding and projecting the evolution of AIDS in the South, they merely had to look back at the persistent and frustrating narrative of syphilis and gonorrhea in the region. For generations, even when public health efforts have stemmed the increase of sexually transmitted diseases in other regions

across the country, the South has been plagued by persistently high rates of syphilis and gonorrhea.

The military conflicts of the first half of the twentieth century helped make syphilis the nemesis of public health officials. World War I caused a seismic "social disruption" that triggered a syphilis epidemic among African Americans. And despite the later efforts of legendary US Surgeon General Dr. Thomas Parran, who was appointed by President Franklin D. Roosevelt in 1936, the epidemic persisted for generations. Through his tireless advocacy, Dr. Parran made it acceptable to use the word *syphilis* in public, although when he first tried to use the term during an interview on the Columbia Broadcasting System, he was muzzled—the show never aired.

Undeterred, Dr. Parran pushed for a "broad-based" publicity campaign to draw attention to the ravages and costs of untreated and unrestrained syphilis on the American public and economy. According to Dr. Parran's estimates, about one in ten Americans would be infected with syphilis during their lifetime. In 1936, long before American boys were preparing to battle Adolf Hitler and the Axis powers overseas, on the home front Dr. Parran convened the National Venereal Disease Conference in Washington, which brought together business, civic, and medical leaders to confront the scourge of syphilis. Thanks largely to the surgeon general's efforts, two years later Congress passed the National Venereal Control Act, creating a nationwide syphilis control plan—essential because state efforts were often sporadic or nonexistent.

While Dr. Parran's 10 percent infection estimates might have been hyperbolic, the advent of World War II opened America's eyes to the true scope of its syphilis infection. More than 170,000 of the 12 million men drafted for military service had to be treated for syphilis before they could be cleared for active duty. Just like it had done to cope with the flu epidemic during World War I, the military created "rapid treatment centers" to deal with syphilis.

War and the massive social and political dislocation of global conflict created a fertile breeding ground for the rapid spread of syphilis. Thus the military brass had to move quickly to prevent a tidal wave of the sexually transmitted disease flooding into America's bedrooms once the fighting stopped. In the twenty-four months from November 1944 to October 1946, as the war wound down and GIs began returning home in massive numbers, more than fifty thousand soldiers, sailors, and airmen were treated for syphilis before they were discharged into civilian life. Despite the government's efforts, in 1947 about 160,000 people were treated for infectious syphilis in America.

The end of the Second World War coincided with the widespread availability of penicillin—a sure cure for syphilis. After the postwar peaks, syphilis rates fell dramatically in the early 1950s. By the mid-'50s only about sixty-five hundred cases of syphilis were being reported annually, which gave public health officials hope that the sexually transmitted disease would be eradicated entirely. But victory would prove elusive. Despite the optimism of the '50s, the "great imitator" launched a comeback. In 1963, public health officials counted more than twenty-two thousand syphilis cases.

The cycle of syphilis is one of epidemic and normalcy, peaks and valleys, in ten-year cycles. At the time of the 1979 Atlanta meeting, public health officials had seen evidence of another emerging epidemic that was mostly in twenty- to twenty-nine-year-old black men in the South. By 1982 that epidemic peaked, infecting black men at astounding rates—thirteen times higher than white men. By then doctors in urban clinics faced a much bigger worry. Scores of gay men were seeking treatment for illnesses that made syphilis look like the common cold.

Initially, the fear of AIDS prompted many to adopt more cautious sexual habits. Syphilis rates dropped as AIDS emerged as the new health crisis. But that trend was temporary. The gain didn't last; just like clockwork, every ten years a syphilis epidemic returns. But in the early 1990s, the demographics had changed. Women were being infected just like the men. One thing didn't change—the color of syphilis. It even became more extreme. The number of black syphilis cases outnumbered white cases by sixty-two to one. The 1990s epidemic wasn't regional; it was national. It began in the West and then struck the South and Northeast before hitting the Midwest. Unlike the previous epidemics, most of the cases were black straight men and women in cities and in the rural South, especially areas where zombielike crack addicts fed their habit by exchanging sex for money or for drugs.

Small towns were the hardest hit. Lancaster, a South Carolina mill town about thirty miles east of Clover, suffered some of the highest syphilis rates in the country as men and women engaged in a never-ending exchange of pleasure and partners. While most of this was sex for pleasure, drugs, or money, between men and women, these communities were also home to a certain level of closeted homosexual activity. Some young men in Clover's black neighborhoods engaged in gay sex for money and pleasure even though they steadfastly identified themselves as straight. They were part of the nascent "down low" culture that flourished in the virulently homophobic African American community. The implications of that historical denial would have far-reaching consequences as the 1980s unfolded.

Prior to the end of World War II, the two most common communicable diseases were measles and syphilis, with gonorrhea a comfortable third. Beginning in 1946, syphilis and gonorrhea switched places, and since 1965 gonorrhea, "the clap," has ranked as the most frequently reported communicable disease in America. During the postwar years, the numbers of reported gonorrhea cases followed a nine-year cycle: from 1948 to 1957 cases dropped at about 5.5 percent annually. This steady decline was followed by a slightly higher rate of increase from 1957 to 1966, after which, thanks largely to the sexual revolution, the number of reported gonorrhea cases doubled to a rate of 12.3 percent per year, until 1975 when health officials reported one million cases. The sharp increases from 1972 to 1975 might have been credited to the inception of the mass screening of women as part of the National Gonorrhea Control Program in 1972. The number of gonorrhea cases plateaued during the three years preceding the 1979 Atlanta conference.

Morgan and his working group would have been very familiar with the numbers as well as the major public health problems caused by STDs and the $1 billion price tag in terms of human suffering, taxpayer dollars, and strain on medical services. In 1976, it cost $770 million to manage and treat gonorrhea, the most common sexually transmitted disease.

The language of those fighting STDs in the late 1970s would later be echoed by those scrambling to contain the plague of HIV/AIDS in the coming decades: "The sexually transmissible disease problem is rooted in apathy and ignorance. Neglect is widespread, dehumanizing and institutionalized" in government and the private sector. "Services to prevent, diagnose and treat sexually transmissible diseases rate low in priority among health budget decision makers, and indeed the general public."

Women and children were the most vulnerable and hardest hit—with sterility, ectopic pregnancy, fetal and infant deaths, and mental retardation. Experts at the conference warned about additional health implications: pelvic inflammatory disease, infant pneumonia, and infant death.

Each year chlamydia caused an estimated fifty thousand eye infections and twenty-four thousand cases of infants with pneumonia. About half a million to one million new cases of herpes simplex were reported. For infected women, having herpes simplex meant more than just the embarrassment of an occasional cold sore on the mouth. Herpes-complicated pregnancies often resulted in miscarriages, stillbirths, or severe neonatal infections. An astounding two-thirds of babies born to mothers with herpes simplex died or were permanently disabled, studies showed.

Sexually transmitted diseases clearly posed a major health care challenge. And Atlanta conference attendees didn't shy away from their task. They even set ambitious goals for the coming decade. They wanted to reduce the incidents of gonorrhea by 30 percent, from one million to seven hundred thousand cases a year. They wanted to reduce the number of primary and secondary syphilis cases from 22,000 to 17,500 a year.

By 1990, they wanted all providers to be able to test for Hepatitis B among gay men; they wanted to reduce the incidents of serious neonatal infection due to herpes and chlamydia by 50 percent. They also recognized the role of education in combating the generational and endemic problem of STDs. By 1990, they wanted each high school student in America to have received a "quality, timely education" in sexual transmitted diseases. That projection might have been politically and culturally naive. Three decades after that historic meeting, sex education has gone backward. Attendees at the Atlanta conference would never have imagined that, with HIV/AIDS ravaging communities, one response from conservative politicians and religious activists would be to promote abstinence-only sex education and to question and denigrate condom use as a method of preventing STDs.

While they might have been naive in terms of their hopes and expectations for youth sex education, the Atlanta group's projection for the future in terms of the evolution of STDs was prescient. "Biologic changes in the organisms that cause sexually transmissible diseases are likely, but unpredictable, as to their occurrences or effects; therefore, they have not been considered."

Those two dozen men and women could not have predicted that, a year later, their colleagues across the country would begin seeing the first signs of a whole new sexually transmissible disease.

Ronald Reagan's election to the White House in 1980 signaled for some a triumph of Americanism and a return of conservatism, a backlash against the cultural excesses of the 1960s and '70s. The former Hollywood actor and California governor entered Washington railing against big government and the Evil Empire, the Soviet Union. While he would be credited with the demise of godless communism and triumphantly ending the Cold War, President Reagan's legacy was tarnished by his administration's "halting and ineffective" response to the outbreak of an unforeseen peril that threatened to decimate the gay and intravenous drug–using populations in America's cities.

As the '80s dawned, America began to recover from the misadventures of the Vietnam War, Watergate, and the Iran hostage crisis. Reagan sought to restore the nation's swagger in confronting all the perceived foreign threats. He ramped up military spending to levels not seen since the height of the wars in Southeast Asia. But the threat wasn't just military. It was invisible except to lab microscopes. It flowed in the veins of men and women. If Reagan's election in 1980 signaled the end of free love and license, then the debt had come due. America's liberalization of attitudes toward sex, gay and straight, and the burgeoning drug culture demoralized inner cities and black neighborhoods. But things were about to get worse. Before 1980, the most painful consequence of an unprotected sexual encounter was the clap or syphilis. It was nothing that a few tablets or a penicillin injection couldn't cure. But the coming decade brought unprecedented perils for the sexually careless and the promiscuous.

Dr. Joel Weisman was a private physician in 1980 when he saw three gay patients in his California practice. The young men all displayed symptoms of what would soon be called gay-related immunodeficiency syndrome, an illness that made previously healthy young gay men vulnerable to a host of deadly opportunistic diseases. Weisman then referred two of the men to Dr. Martin Gottlieb, an immunologist at the University of California at Los Angeles. The following year, Weisman and Gottlieb cowrote a report of the cases and what they saw. Their paper appeared on June 5, 1981, in *Morbidity and Mortality Weekly Report*, published by the CDC almost two years to the day after that major conference on sexually transmitted diseases. The Weisman-Gottlieb document was the first report on AIDS in American medical literature. Over the next twelve months, the media was flooded with accounts of this new plague attacking the mostly white, gay communities in New York City, San Francisco, and Los Angeles.

Physicians and medical researchers struggled to understand the new illness, which wasted its victims, making them vulnerable to rare cancers and pneumonia. They struggled to understand how the disease was transmitted from one human to the next and to develop protocols to help people protect themselves from the deadly new illness.

Scientists would later identify a type of chimpanzee in West Africa as the source of HIV infection in humans. The virus most likely jumped to humans when they hunted these chimpanzees for meat and came into contact with their infected blood. Over several years, the virus slowly spread across Africa and later into other parts of the world. But that knowledge would come much later.

First there were the most pressing questions: Was it a gay disease? And if so, what was it about their lifestyle that made homosexual men so susceptible to the infection? What were the risks to the general population? Once someone was infected, was there a cure?

A year after CDC scientists and researchers in Atlanta began to grapple with the mysterious new illness, about two hundred miles away in Charleston, South Carolina, physicians began to encounter their first patients displaying symptoms that were the harbinger of the coming plague.

6

THE AIDS DOCTOR

It was a typical day in late May 1982. The last blooms still hung onto the azaleas. In Charleston, tourists, like fireflies at night, had descended on the Holy City for the start of the sixth annual Spoleto Festival of the Arts. But Dr. Robert Ball Jr. had more on his mind than symphony orchestras and classical music performances. As he prepared to see patients at his infectious disease clinic in Charleston's West Ashley neighborhood, his phone rang. A family practice physician called seeking an infectious disease consultation for a desperately ill patient.

As an infectious disease specialist, Dr. Ball had grown accustomed to such pleas for help, doctors referring strange cases of tropical diseases to him for care. In less than a decade of medical practice he had developed the reputation of being something of a storm chaser of the infectious diseases that surfaced in the Low Country of South Carolina, an area characterized by viciously hot and humid summers, extensive marshes, and, of course, mosquitoes.

The physician on the other end of the phone line had admitted his patient to St. Francis Xavier Hospital for observation. He was at a loss to determine what ailed the young white man. Without hesitation, Dr. Ball promised to see the patient that day. It was a short drive from his office to the hospital, which had been founded by the Sisters of Charity of Our Lady of Mercy in 1882. When Dr. Ball walked into the private hospital room, he saw a patient who looked to be in his late teens or early twenties. He quickly learned that for several weeks the patient had been suffering from high fevers and swollen lymph nodes. A chicken pox–like rash covered his entire body. Lesions pockmarked his frame, with open, raw sores draining clear fluid. Herpes-like lesions covered his genitals and perineum, the area between his scrotum and anus. On close examination, Ball also noticed that the man had thrush, a yeast infection of the mouth that doctors would later associate closely with being HIV positive.

The young man's swollen lymph nodes signaled trouble. His herpes clearly had been contracted sexually; another disease might have been lurking inside him for several years before trashing his immune system. The symptoms had become too obvious to ignore. Whatever the reason, his health was deteriorating rapidly. "It was the worst case of genital herpes I had ever seen," Dr. Ball says. "Normally, genital herpes doesn't spread throughout your body. In his case, it did."

Thankfully, Dr. Ball determined, the patient didn't have the pneumocystis carinii pneumonia (PCP) or the cancers that physicians had quickly discovered were common among people with AIDS. Of more immediate concern was his extremely low white blood cell count. "There were a number of other lab abnormalities that indicated a systemic infection that was probably viral," Dr. Ball recalls, speaking with an even, genteel southern inflection that could have come straight out of a Pat Conroy novel.

In addition to his private practice, Dr. Ball also taught at the Medical University of South Carolina (MUSC), his alma mater, and knew the lab staff of the huge facility. After he examined the patient, he immediately ordered additional blood tests and further analysis of the man's white blood cells. When the patient's MUSC lab tests came back a week later, they showed an extremely low number of what are now called CD4 lymphocytes. Back then they were called OKT3 lymphocytes. Having low CD4 cell numbers increases the risk of opportunistic infections, leaving an individual as vulnerable as a battleship floating on the high seas without guns. Simple pneumonia could be as lethal as the bubonic plague. Troubled by the initial test results, Dr. Ball ordered more tests. As he awaited the results, he ran through all the possibilities. Little did he know that fateful doctor-patient encounter in St. Francis Hospital on that spring day would turn his comfortable, white, middle-class world upside down, change the course of his professional and personal life, and shake long-held political and spiritual beliefs, transforming him from a white southern Barry Goldwater conservative to that rarest of species, a white southern progressive.

Robert Ball's links to Charleston and the Low Country are as deep and as storied as the region itself. His ancestors first settled on the land when South Carolina was still a colony, more than 320 years ago. The pages of the telephone book are peppered with Balls. He served as president of the Society of First Families of South Carolina, a genealogical organization that documents and celebrates the history of the earliest colonial settlers.

Young Robert grew up in the West Ashley section of Charleston. He played football in high school but was never great at it. His passion was books. He spent hours locked away in his bedroom devouring science books. After high school, unlike many South Carolina blue bloods, he didn't head west for the University of South Carolina in Columbia or even Clemson upstate. Robert remained closer to home. He drove less than half an hour to the College of Charleston, where he studied biology and chemistry. To no one's surprise, he wanted to be a doctor.

In college, Robert, an avid boater, helped form the school's first sailing team. He dabbled in Republican politics and a lot of campus life. His old college yearbooks showed that Robert also was involved with at least four campus organizations each year. He led a Charleston chapter of the John Birch Society, a group that was founded in 1958 by former candy industry executive Robert Welsh, who spouted an ultraconservative brand of pseudo-Christian anticommunism, nationalism, and antiglobalism. John Birch Society members called for the repeal of the federal income tax on constitutional grounds, sought the abolition of the Federal Reserve and the United Nations, and viewed the civil rights movement as the vanguard of a communist plot. In 1964, like most other John Birch Society members, Ball supported Barry Goldwater. The conservative Arizona senator had lost to Nixon in the 1960 Republican primaries but prevailed against moderates

Governor Nelson A. Rockefeller of New York and Governor William Scranton of Pennsylvania before being trounced by the incumbent president, Lyndon Johnson, in 1964.

Two years later, after he graduated from the College of Charleston, Ball followed a path he seemed genetically bred to pursue. He drove across town and enrolled at what was then the Medical College of South Carolina, an institution whose desks, chairs, and labs were stained with the sweat of his forebears. Ball is descended from a line of physicians seven generations deep. His great-grandfather was a doctor; a number of great-uncles were too. One uncle was a physician; another, Benjamin M. Martin, was chief radiology technician at MUSC for over two decades. Both grandfathers were doctors, and his paternal grandfather, Dr. James Austin Ball, was the medical school's first professor of infectious diseases, then called tropical medicine, at the turn of the century. His maternal grandfather, Dr. Thomas Hutson Martin, graduated from the College of Medicine in 1919 at age nineteen before launching a long and distinguished career as a physician and surgeon in Charleston. Dr. Martin was a longtime member of the Charleston County Board of Health and an assistant professor of surgery at the medical school. He retired from practicing medicine in 1951. Later, Ball would donate Dr. Martin's class ring to the medical school's Waring Historical Library.

The oldest medical school in the Deep South, the Medical College of South Carolina was founded in 1824 and kept its name largely intact for 145 years. But by the time Ball donned his cap and gown to accept his medical degree in 1970, the college had been renamed the Medical University of South Carolina. He helped put himself through medical school by working days as an anatomy instructor and nights in the MUSC microbiology lab. For his medical internship, he drove 470 miles west on Interstate 20 to the University of Alabama–Birmingham, which was located in a city that had come to symbolize southern white resistance to the struggle for black civil rights. But less known at the time was that its hospital was a vital training ground for infectious disease specialists. Later it would be home to several pioneers in the fight against HIV and AIDS.

Ball began his medical internship, now called a residency, in Birmingham the same year George Wallace returned in triumph to the governor's mansion for a second four-year term. Wallace was still a rabid segregationist who opposed equal rights for people of color. The young Ball admired Wallace's uncompromising segregationist anti–civil rights platform. That was before his epiphany; that was before AIDS, before he saw firsthand the machinery of white privilege and southern prejudice, once reserved exclusively for people of color, unleashed on white gay men with a deadly, demoralizing new sickness.

Wallace and his politics of derision appealed to Ball at his deepest core. On holidays he drove east to Charleston, proudly showing off the Wallace bumper stickers on his car. Those stickers multiplied as Wallace ran again for the presidency in 1972 after his failed bid in 1968.

Parents, classmates, and friends weren't surprised by Ball's affinity for Goldwater and Wallace. Like most well-off southern white men, Ball grew up in a very politically conservative family, even though their hometown, Charleston, was becoming increasingly liberal. His family was Republican, the kind who scoffed at northeastern Republican moderates. Ball, still a fervent anticommunist, spent years licking his wounds after Senator Goldwater's 1964 defeat at the hands of LBJ.

That decisive election was to have a direct impact on Ball's fate. After his re-election, Johnson escalated America's involvement in Vietnam. For the next six years, rural southern boys and inner city kids in their teens and early twenties were drafted and shipped, weapons in hand, to the jungles of Southeast Asia. Ball's medical internship only delayed the inevitable. The draft board gave him permission to finish his training. Sooner or later the army would beckon. As the war in Vietnam dragged on, even white boys of privilege couldn't avoid doing their share in the increasingly unpopular war. The summer Americans first heard about the Pentagon Papers, when protestors in Washington tried to bring the federal government to its knees, Ball, now at the end of his internship in Birmingham, received the long-feared letter—a direct order to report to the draft board in Charleston. Days later, he walked into the draft board office in Charleston and swore his allegiance to defend the country. He was lucky. The army wanted to send him as an orthopedic surgeon to the combat zone in Vietnam, where American GIs needed able surgeons to repair the damage wrought by Vietcong booby traps. But his skills did not lie in the operating room. "You want me with a pen in my hand, not a scalpel," he joked years later. "No wonder we were losing over there."

Ball spent his two-year tour of duty working as medical director of the emergency department at the massive William Beaumont Army Medical Center complex in El Paso, Texas, which serves neighboring Fort Bliss. By the time he was honorably discharged in 1973, the end was in sight for the US military involvement in Vietnam, but the country had just begun a spiral toward another prolonged political crisis—Watergate.

Ball returned home as expected to Charleston, where for the next two years he pursued an internal medicine residency, followed by a twenty-four-month infectious diseases and immunology fellowship at his alma mater, MUSC. Ball was hardwired not just to study medicine but also to hunt infectious diseases, just like his paternal grandfather, Dr. Ball, who in the early 1900s taught dermatology and tropical diseases. Graveyards in the South are filled with children and young people victimized by smallpox, yellow fever, and cholera. Sexually transmitted diseases, especially syphilis and gonorrhea, ran rampant through the poor sectors, especially the black population. While he was serving in the army, Ball contracted viral meningitis, a relatively common but rarely serious infection of the fluid in the spinal cord and surrounding the brain. Viral meningitis and other infectious diseases fascinated Ball. After he was discharged from the military, he hoped to pursue a specialty that offered the daily challenge of trying to cure people with the new and exciting antibiotics being introduced daily rather than deal with terminal conditions like cancer. But the good Lord had other ideas.

His long journey to becoming a physician complete, Ball opened a private practice in the West Ashley section of Charleston in 1977. Jimmy Carter had been elected to the White House a year earlier. America was still struggling to rediscover its self-confidence. While he built his fledgling practice, Ball taught part time at MUSC, honoring his family legacy.

While Dr. Ball taught infectious diseases, elsewhere in the massive MUSC complex a high-cheekboned black woman, Annie Mae Pegram, cheerfully endured the pricks and prods from physicians testing new cancer drugs. It's unlikely that their paths ever crossed, but fate conspired to ensure that AIDS, the disease that dominated Dr. Ball's private and public medical career, would also shape the life and cause the early death of Annie Mae's youngest daughter, Carolyn.

As a young boy, Robert Ball was always an obsessive reader, a habit that remained into adulthood. When he became a physician, he simply changed the hours accordingly. On most weeknights he lay awake long past midnight reading medical literature on the latest infectious disease threats invading America. One of those nights in 1981, even as his friends and colleagues wined and dined at one of Charleston's frequent cocktail parties, Ball read a report from the CDC alerting physicians around the country about a deadly condition that had mysteriously appeared in five young gay men in Los Angeles.

After five years in practice, Dr. Ball had gained a reputation for being on the cutting edge of infectious disease surveillance. Doctors sent him patients stricken with strange and undiagnosed illnesses. He gained some notoriety for being the first physician in the Palmetto state to diagnose Legionnaires' disease, an illness caused by a type of bacteria called *Legionella*, which earned its name in 1976 when many people who attended an American Legion convention in Philadelphia fell ill with a pneumonia-like lung infection. During this exciting period early in his practice, Ball was among the first physicians in the state to diagnose a patient with toxic shock syndrome, a condition caused by *Staphylococcus aureus* bacteria and initially linked to a particular type of high-absorbency tampons. Toxic shock syndrome can attack a patient who has any type of staph infection, such as pneumonia, an abscess, a skin or wound infection, a blood infection, or the bone infection osteomyelitis.

By May 1982, when Dr. Ball saw his first patient with suspicious symptoms of what was initially called gay-related immunodeficiency disease, public health experts knew the condition was not just confined to gay men—it was also infecting heterosexuals who had received blood transfusions and health care workers accidentally pricked by contaminated needles.

Much had been learned about the immune system prior to 1980, but since the arrival of HIV/AIDS, researchers have learned so much more. Necessity accelerated the learning curve. One breakthrough was the discovery that CD4 helper lymphocytes did marvelous things. They served as what Dr. Anthony S. Fauci, director of the National Institute of Allergy and Infectious Diseases, called "the conductor of the immune system's orchestra," coordinating dozens of immune system cells to deal with pathogens—viruses, fungi, or bacteria—that are potentially deadly foreign microscopic invaders. But in 1982, one year into the battle to slow the spread of AIDS and save those made deathly ill by this strange disease, physicians were like pilots flying in the dark without navigation equipment. They played hunches. Sometimes they guessed right, but often they were wrong.

Dr. Ball took a week to diagnose Patient No. 1, as he took to calling his first AIDS patient. Ball knew about his low T-4 or CD4 lymphocytes, and when the lab tests returned, the physician had few options. That made his job easier. He prescribed the antiviral medicine Acyclovir, now sold under the trade name Zovirax, via intravenous drip for three weeks. During the third week, the patient's herpes had cleared up and his fever downgraded. Unlike many AIDS patients, the young man had good insurance to pay for his lengthy hospital stay.

Faced with an illness far more complex than any of the infectious diseases he had ever encountered, Dr. Ball contacted his colleagues at CDC in Atlanta and Dr. Eric Brenner, who worked in Columbia with the South Carolina Department of Health and Environmental Control (DHEC) surveillance section. Dr. Ball also spoke with several other colleagues to confirm that what he was seeing was indeed the new condition they had diagnosed on the East and West Coasts. Initially, physicians and researchers had dubbed the illness GRID—gay-related immunodeficiency disease—because the overwhelming majority of the early cases were diagnosed among gay men. But it didn't take long for CDC epidemiologists to realize that this disease, which they renamed AIDS in 1982, was also infecting blood transfusion recipients, heterosexuals, and intravenous drug users. This was no mere disease; it was a syndrome, a medical term used to describe a cluster of symptoms and signs for which at the time you may or may not know the cause. And researchers were still guessing about what caused this illness.

"Gay sex and IV drug use spread AIDS more efficiently than heterosexual sex," Dr. Ball said. Patient No. 1 had a complicated sexual history. After some prodding, he admitted to having had both gay and straight sex, with numerous partners, since he was a teenager. That was at least five years of sexual activity that put him at risk. The man contracted the infection through sexual intercourse several years before his health had deteriorated into full-blown AIDS. "I'm reminded of a joke," Dr. Ball said with a chuckle. "Promiscuous is defined as anybody who has one more sex partner than you or me."

As the young man responded well to treatment during his second week of hospitalization, the MUSC laboratory tests showed the patient had extremely low lymphocytes, a condition that physicians later began to see in people with AIDS. "They had never seen anything like that," Dr. Ball says.

Lab director Dr. Mariano LaVia had been Ball's good friend since the late 1970s. The two men spoke often. Both knew that this new phenomenon had surfaced in patients and was being called acquired immune deficiency syndrome—acquired because the patients weren't born with it and because their immune system was now deficient. In the summer of 1982, scientists and researchers already knew that HTLV-I and HTLV-II existed. Those two strains caused a slight immune deficiency but nothing like this. It wasn't until 1984 that researchers correctly identified the virus and renamed it human immunodeficiency virus (HIV).

With aggressive antiherpes treatment, Patient No. 1 rallied. His case caught the attention of CDC researchers and private labs. Soon afterward, several labs, including a Research Triangle Park, North Carolina, outfit, expressed interest in studying whether acquired immune deficiency syndrome was transmitted by blood. They came calling for some samples from

Patient No. 1. "They wanted more than a tube," Ball recalls. "They wanted a half pint."

The young man agreed to donate his infected blood. Organon-Teknika, based in Research Triangle Park, near Raleigh, was one of the first labs in the country to use antibody-antigen testing for various viruses. Scientists for Organon-Teknika reported that Patient No. 1 had extremely high concentrations of antibodies in his blood. They wanted more samples to study. "They called back very excited," Dr. Ball.

Patient No. 1 was so relieved that his fever had subsided, his sores had healed, and his various other ailments had improved that he eagerly agreed to donate a pint of blood every few months. The labs paid him a token sum for his trouble. "It wasn't much; it was just enough to make it worth his while," says Dr. Ball.

By the end of 1983, Patient No. 1's blood was one of a few national positive samples against which other patient samples were compared. In scientific lab jargon, he was the positive control. That lasted for two years, until 1985 when Organon-Teknika devised a blood test that US Department of Health and Human Services desperately needed to help screen the nation's blood supply. By then, scores of blood transfusion recipients, including tennis great Arthur Ashe, had been fatally infected. The primary concern from CDC epidemiologists was the safety of the nation's blood supply. Millions of pints of blood destined for America's emergency rooms and operating tables were at risk of being infected by HIV. Thousands of lives were in danger. Federal officials could only protect the blood supply if they had a reliable blood test. That test confirmed the presence of antibodies in a patient's blood, not the virus: the occurrence of the antibody proves the presence of the virus.

As part of his treatment regimen, Dr. Ball prescribed Acyclovir to take whenever his herpes flared up. The young man tried to curb his sexual activity, but he later confessed to slipping a few times. Chastened, the patient tried being socially responsible. He volunteered at the local health department to provide educational programs in the community. He tried to use his bad situation for public good, but he didn't want his identity known. People would see his face, but he didn't want his name published.

The encounter with that first young, gay white man suffering from AIDS proved to be a turning point in Dr. Ball's medical career. Dr. Ball calls it a gradual awakening. But in retrospect, it was no less than an epiphany in his social and political evolution. After May 1982, his practice changed.

Ball worked eighteen hours a day treating the mostly gay white men who came knocking at his door, their bodies racked by pneumonia and other diseases, desperately seeking his help, hoping that he could prolong if not save their lives. This was what he had dreamed of in medical school—a practice that would be emotionally and professionally fulfilling. He was making a difference in the lives of those he treated. But these patients were mostly disabled and jobless because of their debilitating illness. Most of them had no health insurance and only meager savings. Many felt abandoned by their families. These patients were a money-losing proposition for a private doctor. They didn't pay their bills, and insurance companies usually denied coverage claiming pre-existing conditions, Ball said. That was compounded when Ball's paying patients became offended by his treatment of AIDS patients. One-third of his private practice patients left him. Some said they didn't want to share the same waiting area and examination room with "those people." Many switched doctors without saying a word. After a while, it became painfully obvious why they stopped coming to see him. He was the AIDS doctor—a pariah in his own community.

However, some of his patients were polite about the whole thing. They just weren't comfortable coming to see the AIDS doctor, they said. They didn't want anyone to suspect them of having AIDS; they didn't want to risk catching the disease. He could understand that. There was so much about AIDS even doctors and medical professionals didn't understand. And his medical partners were no exception. They refused to take calls from his AIDS patients. "I don't like being in the same room with those people," one doctor said. Some lacked the medical knowledge, but others felt uneasy caring for gay men. "I don't want to treat them," they said.

For Ball, this most exhilarating and emotionally rewarding period of his medical career was also the most financially frustrating. In 1986 Ball found himself going solo, working about a hundred hours a week, seeing patients from morning until late at night. Despite all the hard work and long hours, he slipped deep into debt. One year he took home $18,000, a paltry sum for a respectable physician in affluent Charleston. With the long hours and mounting financial strain, his marriage, like his practice, suffered.

He and his wife soon divorced. The bank foreclosed on his house. All he owned was his car and several pieces of furniture. He moved into an apartment. In the end, he was forced to sell the practice to pay off his debts and pay his staff. Dr. Ball was only forty-two.

He was fortunate. His contacts in the medical community helped him get a part-time job with the Department of Health and Environmental Control, the state's public health agency that runs a network of public clinics and monitors the state's health. Ball moved into an apartment in Columbia, the state capital, and enrolled at the University of South Carolina to pursue a master's degree in public health. He also enrolled in a preventive medical fellowship. For a blue-blooded Charleston physician, it was a stunning fall from grace. But the call to fight AIDS demands a long-term commitment. Ball's move to Columbia gave him a statewide platform to deal with the illness that had destroyed so many lives. His move to public service was also a major detour from the affluence brought by private medical practice, but for Ball it was also the fulfillment of his family legacy. After all, hadn't his ancestors been known for their work in public health? He was a key player in South Carolina's medical hierarchy when, in July 1994, he learned of the death of Patient No. 1. He had survived AIDS for more than a decade.

And Ball? Working for the Department of Health and Environmental Control, Dr. Ball led the state task force that developed South Carolina's Ryan White program, the main federal mechanism for financing the fight against AIDS and HIV. Later he returned to his hometown, Charleston, to work as a state health department infectious disease consultant and epidemiologist with a focus on emerging infectious diseases and bioterrorism. He lives in his boyhood home on Charleston Harbor with his wife, a retired public health nurse. His personal and professional journey had come full circle.

7

DR. MICHAEL WATSON

Even as Robert Ball's private practice unraveled under the weight of the stigma of AIDS, eighty miles west, in Bamberg, located in the heart of South Carolina's Black Belt, a small-town physician, Dr. Michael Watson, found new purpose with the arrival of this unprecedented illness.

Dr. Watson came from an earlier generation of physicians, yet he had much in common with Ball. Both traced their family ancestry deep into the roots of southern soil. Both loved to read from an early age. By the time he reached the seventh grade, Mickey, as his father called him, had read every book in his school library. Both shared the infectious disease physician's sense of mission. Like Ball, Watson had served in the military during wartime, although he was much closer to the fighting—he fought in the South Pacific during World War II. Watson also studied medicine at the Medical College of South Carolina almost two decades before Ball arrived.

Watson was born in a red brick house in Ridge Spring, Saluda County, South Carolina, on January 15, 1926, the same day the New York Yankees sold Wally Pipp to the Cincinnati Reds for $7,500. Pipp, baseball fans know, secured a place in the annals of America's pastime after a twenty-two-year-old named Lou Gehrig replaced him in the Yankees lineup and never relinquished the spot for a record-setting 2,130 games.

The Watsons lived on about one hundred acres of farmland that had been given to the family by Kings George II and George III of England before the Revolutionary War.

Watson's well-to-do father, Joseph Calhoun "Cal" Watson, grew cotton and asparagus for the markets; he cultivated sugarcane and other vegetables for the dinner table. But the success of the modern southern farm was always tied to events on Wall Street and distant capitals. The stock market crash of 1929 and the ensuing Great Depression turned the circumstances of the Watson household upside down. Cotton sold for a nickel a pound, but the boll weevil ensured that there wasn't much cotton to weigh. To stave off ruin, Cal Watson went to work for a local bank. When that bank failed, Cal Watson went to work for the Seed Loan, a Depression-era agency of the US Department of Agriculture, which sent him to work in Kentucky. He was gone from 1933 to 1940. He came home for a week at Christmas and a week during the summer. In his absence, Watson's mother, Aurelia Cunningham Watson, who was raised among the textile mills in the upstate town of Greer, had to fend for herself. While Watson began life as upper middle class, hard times brought the family low. At one point the Saluda County sheriff threatened to sell the Watson farm for failure to pay taxes. His mother begged a relative for help. In his unpublished autobiography, Watson recalled an incident that would have been eerily familiar to Tricia Ann Starr and those who grew up in Annie Mae Pegram's household. The owner of the local telephone company called one day and requested payment on the Watson's past due account. Young Mickey, who could hear only one side of the conversation, heard his mother say, "I intend to pay you when I can, but if you can't wait, just come and take the telephone out."

"He never came," Watson recalls.

Aurelia Watson operated the farm with the help of the black foreman and more than half a dozen farm hands who drove the six mules to plow the land. That the farmstead survived was largely because of the loyalty of the laborers, who stayed while many of their friends and relatives left the South.

The Great Northern Migration in the years before and after World War I jeopardized southern farmers' cheap labor supply. Legions of black laborers fled Ku Klux Klan intimidation, Jim Crow oppression, and joblessness due to mechanization and headed for the industrial cities of the North and Midwest. In 1926, the year Watson was born, whites in South Carolina became a majority statewide for the first time since 1810. Eight decades later, even as Saluda County boasted a white majority, Ridge Spring, his hometown, remained over 60 percent black.

Young Mickey—his father insisted that no one call him Mike—helped on the farm, but his heart was elsewhere. Farm work came more naturally to Joe. He loved to toil alongside the black men, women, and child laborers who worked on the farm. He even became a farmer. But the proximity to the rigors of Southern farm life exposed Mickey to the poverty, sickness, pain, and tragedy of black workers. At the same time, he came to appreciate their loyalty, good humor, generosity, and trustworthiness. That experience fostered a deep empathy with the black people who worked on his family's farm. It marked him for life.

The day the Japanese bombed Pearl Harbor in December 1941, Watson, a tenth-grader in high school, was hitchhiking home from visiting his older brother Joe at Clemson, then an all-male military college. A generous motorist picked him up in Saluda, and as the two drove home toward Ridge Spring, they listened to the news of the attack on the car radio.

Like most young men of his generation, Mickey wanted to enlist. But he was too young to sign up and needed his parents' permission. They refused. As a dutiful son, he bided his time; in the fall of 1943, still only seventeen, he enrolled in Clemson to study engineering. But he knew the Saluda County draft board awaited him as soon as he turned eighteen. He preferred to enlist. He tried to sign up for naval flight school, but they rejected him because of what Watson called a pigeon chest deformity—he wouldn't fit in the flight harness. Soon afterward, Watson enlisted in the Marine Corps. With his high IQ, Watson was assigned to electronics school to study radar. After basic training on Parris Island, South Carolina, he spent about ten months at Camp Lejeune, North Carolina, before shipping overseas to Guam in the South Pacific, where he manned a searchlight battery until VE Day in 1945. Watson heard news of the atomic bomb being dropped on Hiroshima, Japan, while he was aboard a troop ship headed back to the United States to enroll in officer candidate school.

After the Marine Corps honorably discharged him in 1946, Watson took immediate advantage of the GI Bill of Rights. He returned to Clemson and hurried to make up for time lost during his enlistment. He initially considered becoming an electrical engineer but switched to pre-med after one year. In 1949, after just three years at Clemson, he headed down to the Low Country to what was then the Medical College of South Carolina in Charleston. Uncle Sam paid Mickey's Clemson and medical school tuition and gave him a modest living allowance.

For four years, Watson studied medicine, including infectious diseases—kidney infections, sore throats, gonorrhea, and syphilis—ailments that afflicted many of the poor people, black and white, of his small county. Then he traveled north for his one-year internship at the Maumee Valley Hospital in Toledo, Ohio. With his talent and military credentials, Watson could easily have opened a lucrative private practice in Cleveland, Cincinnati, Indianapolis, or some other major Midwestern city. Instead his heart lay at home in the South. The young physician looked for the most medically underserved area in a fifty-mile radius from his hometown, where his parents still lived. He settled in Bamberg in 1954.

While being a doctor certainly gave Watson social status, he returned to the South at an uncertain time. In the summer of 1954, the US Supreme Court ruled that school segregation was illegal. State authorities throughout the South threatened to resist the court's ruling. Bamberg County, with its majority black population and minority white leadership, might explode if local authorities mishandled desegregation. But Watson was undeterred. He served on the school board during those trying times. Service was a compulsion for him. Bamberg was always a very poor county. His calling was to serve the poor. He would never be one of those wealthy, big-city doctors. He recognized that when he was in medical school in Charleston treating patients with maggots crawling on their flesh. He knew that when he treated children with polio during his internship in Toledo. "It was a big turning point when I realized that my place was the place of a server," he says. "I was not a grandiose physician. I was a servant of the people."

Professionally, he timed his arrival in Bamberg perfectly. A local physician had died several months earlier, and his office sat empty and unused in downtown Bamberg. Watson rented the office from the doctor's widow and set out to equip it. His private practice, Michael C. Watson, MD, opened in 1954, and for the next half a century Watson was the iconic small-town physician who sought to heal the physical, sexual, and social ills that afflicted the residents of his small county. First he hired a secretary and a nurse. During the 1950s, most Southern rural women delivered babies at home attended by a midwife. Watson wanted to offer them a safer alternative. He bought a table so he could deliver babies in his office, which in keeping with the norms of Jim Crow segregation was outfitted with two waiting rooms—one black, one white.

He split his time between his private clinic and Bamberg County Memorial Hospital, which had opened its doors in 1952. Watson began as a staff physician and later rose to become medical director. At that time, Bamberg Hospital operated without a full-time emergency room physician, so people rousted Watson out of his bed almost nightly to attend to someone who had fallen ill at home or an injured motorist.

"I never missed a house call, except one time," he says. On that occasion, the phone rang at three o'clock one morning, a woman needing medical care. So Watson climbed out of bed, dressed, and followed her exact directions to her house. But he couldn't find it. Southern hospitality is scarce at 3:00 AM. "People don't take kindly to someone knocking on their door at that time of the morning," he says. "No one would tell me how to find her."

Many of Watson's routine house calls turned into emergency baby deliveries. Husbands and soon-to-be fathers played the game well. It was much cheaper for their wives to give birth at home than in Watson's specially equipped office.

"Can you come to see my wife? She's bad off," they'd tell him over the phone.

"Is she pregnant?" Watson would ask. The men almost always answered no, but when he drove up to the house, he usually found a woman in labor and ready to deliver. But even as he was busy delivering babies in the shacks and farmhouses around Bamberg, Dr. Watson never missed his special deliveries. In September 1956, he married Mary Carolyn Tatum, a Low Country woman who taught school in Columbia. When they returned from their honeymoon, she wanted to talk about having children. She wanted six.

"That's all right, but I am thirty years old," he told her. "If we have one in two years and one every two years after that, how old would I be when the sixth one came?"

Their first child arrived the day before their first anniversary and, like clockwork, the next five children followed every year and a half afterward: three girls and three boys. Nine years separated the first from the last. They grew up to be three physicians, two attorneys, and one college professor.

Perhaps Watson felt driven by the demands of feeding and clothing six young children; maybe his passion for medicine just pushed him, and it was inevitable that Watson would venture into public health medicine. So many of his patients could barely afford to pay. Many, he knew, sought care at the Bamberg County Health Department downtown.

Poor folks in Bamberg, like in many poor, small, rural communities such as Clover, went to the public health clinic for treatment. They'd walk up to the window, and a staff member would inquire why the person needed treatment. "Most patients were very poor," he says. "The health department took care of indigent patients who couldn't afford a private doctor."

In 1966 he became the Bamberg County Health Department medical director, a post he held for over a quarter of a century. Clinic staff treated a nonstop parade of patients seeking care for syphilis and gonorrhea in addition to the usual maladies that afflict poor country folk. "Gonorrhea was too common," Watson says.

He usually dispensed antibiotics to men with gonorrhea, but women who had no symptoms were frequently ignorant of their condition and often went untreated for years, wreaking untold damage on their reproductive systems. That changed, however, with the introduction of cultures to diagnose and treat those infected with gonorrhea. After Watson read about the use of cultures to test women for gonorrhea, he approached the state health department in Columbia about putting the pilot program in the

Bamberg County Health Department, the main source of nonemergency medical care for the hundreds of poor uninsured men, women, and children in the area.

Women who came for a gynecological examination were automatically cultured for gonorrhea. Dr. Watson expanded the program by getting private physicians to agree to culture their patients at the Health Department's expense. That was one of the first public STD screening programs in the state and became a model for other rural South Carolina communities and a precursor for dealing with AIDS.

While working at the county clinic part-time, Dr. Watson began to notice much more than the sore throats, kidney infections, and STDs. He observed a pattern of strange illnesses he had never encountered in his more than thirty years of being a small-town doctor. "These HIV positive people had all kinds of weird infections," Watson says. "These were unusual infections, and we didn't know anything about how to treat them, except what was in books."

Around the same time, Watson's old friend Margaret Jenkins first encountered people grieving and dying of AIDS in Rock Hill. That was 1989, eight years after doctors on the West Coast first saw what would be known as AIDS and more than six years since Dr. Robert Ball had encountered his first case less than two hours away in Charleston.

Soon afterward, Watson convened a staff meeting at Bamberg County Memorial Hospital with the nurses and the eight staff doctors. He had a major announcement. "I plan to start an AIDS clinic at the health department," he told them. "If you have any AIDS patients, you can send them to me." Watson didn't have to wait long for a reaction.

"You must be crazy," one young and usually respectful doctor blurted out. That skepticism extended far beyond Watson's colleagues and the Bamberg County line. Some at the headquarters of the Department of Health and Environmental Control in Columbia doubted Watson's clinic could work. They envisioned that in a small town where everyone knew one another, where secrets were open and the chances for stigma were greatest, no one would visit an AIDS clinic for treatment.

Among the skeptics was Dr. Robert Ball, who had made a name for himself as the first physician to identify an AIDS patient in South Carolina and whose private practice was destroyed by the stigma surrounding AIDS. From the beginning of his public service tenure, Ball worked alongside state epidemiologist Dr. Eric Brenner and state STD/HIV program director Lynda Kettinger to "establish the state's reporting system" and direct the state's long-delayed response to AIDS. At the time, Ball strongly doubted that an HIV clinic could work in the small-town county health department.

"He thought it was too complex an issue," Watson says. "It wouldn't work in a clinic in such a small community health office. I knew it could." In addition to his private practice, Watson worked several hours a day as director of the Bamberg County Health Department from 1966 to 1992. In the mid-'90s, he became the clinic physician at the Changes Clinic for HIV and AIDS at the Bamberg Health Department.

In a small town like Bamberg, where everyone knew one another's business before it happened, patient privacy could have been an issue. "We didn't have a problem keeping patients' information confidential," Watson says. "We insisted that the staff be ethical. It worked out."

When he admitted the first man with AIDS to the Bamberg hospital, Watson didn't know how the nurses would treat the patient because of fear. It didn't take long to find out. Soon after the patient entered the hospital ward, one worried nurse walked up to Dr. Watson with a question her colleagues no doubt wished they had the courage to ask.

"What am I going to have to do to keep from catching it?" she asked, her face lined with concern. The word *it* dropped off her lips as if she were afraid that even referring to AIDS made it contagious. In response Dr. Watson leaned over and whispered mischievously into her ear, "You don't have sex with him." The nurse burst out laughing loud enough for the whole ward to hear. That moment of levity broke the tension and put the nursing staff at ease. "They were really good to him," Watson says. "They were very compassionate and wonderful."

Watson's pioneering work with AIDS was not unprecedented. He had broken new medical ground before. Early in his medical practice, after he spent long hours treating his patients for diabetes and high blood pressure, he had established a hypertension clinic, one of the first in the Southeast. In cosmopolitan Charleston, Dr. Ball's medical practice failed because non-AIDS patients who didn't want to be treated by the "AIDS doc" had other options. In geographically isolated, economically depressed Bamberg, Dr. Watson's patients had little choice.

From the beginning, an infectious disease doctor in Columbia, Dr. Bosco Postic, offered free long-distance consultations. Whenever Watson encountered an exceptionally difficult case, he called Dr. Postic, who advised him what to do and what to watch out for. Invariably he saw good results. Watson also worked with nurses who willingly treated patients local physicians stoutly refused to see.

Deep in the Bible Belt, it didn't help that so many of the early cases of AIDS were homosexual men. Southerners seemed culturally bred to despise gays. Although he was a man of deep religious faith, Watson didn't share their discomfort. Perhaps his early exposure to black people, the outcast and despised people of his community, prepared him for this assignment.

Watson tells the story of a physician in an adjoining county who sent a middle-aged patient to see a gynecologist in Orangeburg, one of the larger towns close to Bamberg. After the specialist performed a blood test, he discovered the woman was HIV positive. He gave her the bad news, and then he wrote a letter for her to carry to her primary care physician. When she returned to her doctor, she sat in his office while he read the letter from the gynecologist. After the doctor was finished reading, he looked up at the patient. "He told her, 'Get out of my office and never come back,'" Watson says. "It was bad. He turned her off so completely, she didn't seek medical care at all."

Like many AIDS patients in those uncertain days, the woman kept her diagnosis secret. After the patient became deathly ill, a nurse saw her and suggested she visit Dr. Watson at the AIDS clinic. When she showed up, he promptly admitted her to the hospital. The woman had less than a month to live, but her family was ignorant of what was killing her. "Dr. Watson, my children don't know what's wrong with me," she told Watson that day. "I think they should know, and I want you to tell them."

Watson agreed, and the woman summoned her four children to her hospital room the next day. They had no idea their mother was dying of AIDS. "She died two weeks later," Watson says.

Treating people with HIV and AIDS always carried its own risks. One day at the clinic, Watson encountered an HIV-positive patient and her newborn. During that uncertain time, research was unclear on mother-to-child HIV transmission. He decided to test the baby to see if it was infected.

As he described in his unpublished autobiography, the way to draw blood from an infant is different than from an adult. It required the physician or nurse to place the index finger deep in the notch in the front of the lower neck with one hand and hold the syringe and needle in the other hand. Dr. Watson inserted the needle until he could feel the prick of the needle against his index finger. But as he began to withdraw the barrel of the syringe, filling the vacant space with blood, he felt the needle penetrate his rubber glove and his skin. "I'm not sure why; maybe the baby jerked in the hands of the nurse holding it," he recalls.

After he finished drawing the baby's blood and removed his glove, he looked at his index finger. A small drop of blood appeared. His blood had commingled with the baby's. His heart raced. What if it was HIV positive?

Thankfully it wasn't.

8

CAROLYN: THE CRAZY '80S

As the threat of AIDS spread from America's biggest cities in the Northeast and West to the smallest hamlets in the Deep South, Carolyn and her friends in Clover lived in full party mode, oblivious to the perils of easy sex and rampant drug use.

She was petulant; she was strong willed. She was Carolyn. The baby girl of the Pegram clan, she was too young to have known her mother as a vibrant, active woman. But she was old enough to remember the pain of being raised by a mother who was too sick to do all those things little girls love to do with their mothers. And so after Annie Mae died in 1979, Carolyn, just fifteen and essentially an orphan, set out to carve her own way in the world.

She was buxom. Her arms were thick as a young pine sapling, her hips and behind fully formed, each inch protruding outward like an invitation to the men who ogled her as she walked by. She quit junior high school. And just as her dying mother had feared, Carolyn was rootless and unguided in the world. After all, Tricia Ann was married and had three little boys and a husband to care for. She couldn't care for her family and care for Carolyn too. John, the oldest sibling, was also married. He had his own familial responsibilities. Carolyn needed a strong authority figure, someone who could rein in her impetuousness, someone who could provide shelter and comfort in a tough world. That person was supposed to be her father's sister, a woman they called Aunt Ellen. She could take care of Carolyn; she could grab Carolyn before she was gone too far.

But it was already too late. Carolyn had sampled the fast life. She had more than a few sexual partners. She drank. She smoked. Plus Carolyn could never stand Aunt Ellen's rules. Carolyn stayed briefly with Tricia Ann, but she was out of control. She had a reputation. John couldn't take her either. She decided she wanted to live in Newark, New Jersey, with an uncle, so she boarded a Greyhound bus for the eighteen-hour trip north. She stayed for a year in the big city before her uncle, fearing for her life, packed her back south to John.

Carolyn wasn't yet seventeen, but she lived like an adult. All day long she walked back and forth in the neighborhood. She always wore a smile, the kind of smile that undressed bearded, gray-haired men and made them contemplate acts that were probably illegal in every state in the Union. When Carolyn moved in with her brother John for a while, his youngest daughter, Tracy, came to adore Carolyn. But to Tracy's father, Carolyn was a daily nightmare. One day John was walking down the street in the neighborhood and overheard a group of men talking. The men boasted about the previous night's sexual exploits. In turn each described all the things he had done with a woman. Her name was Carolyn. They ignored John, unaware that he was Carolyn's brother. He was a Walker; she was a Pegram. They could not have known that their words fell on a big brother's ears like daggers to an innocent man's heart. He could not fight for his sister. There was no honor to defend, only shame to endure. He walked by in silence, his heart alive with pain. Tears filled his eyes as he walked to the home of Tricia Ann, who by then had moved back to Clover. He stepped inside and wept aloud like a child for his baby sister.

Carolyn's long, dark trip began in the usual places, in the usual ways. She hung around with the men and women who sat under the shade trees in dirt backyards and sipped beer from forty-ounce bottles and swigged cheap rye liquor that made their heads vibrate and let them forget whatever tortured past they were trying to outrun.

Soon the beer and bourbon failed to dull Carolyn's pain. Her older friends had graduated from booze to heroin and crack and had been to rehab and back again. Soon Carolyn's siblings noticed the needle marks on her elbows and her feet, telltale footprints on the dirt road to ruin.

Those were less obvious than the long disappearances. She would be gone without a trace for days on end only to resurface with a smile and an alibi. Carolyn often found herself in abandoned houses, surrounded by strange men and women who shared her insatiable desire for the warm embrace of the drugs she used to dull her senses, quiet bad memories, and help her forget the prick of separation from her mother. "Many days I lay down and I didn't want to get up," Carolyn told me a year or two before her death.

Her life dissolved into an unstoppable merry-go-round of sex, drugs, money, stealing, plotting, and conniving to fill that void inside her. Her appetite for drugs served like a can of gas in the hands of an arsonist. Tricia Ann never saw Carolyn shooting up, but one day she glimpsed a rubber tourniquet, needle, and spoon in Carolyn's pocketbook.

Carolyn also loved the company and attention of grown men, men old enough to be her father. Nothing her sister and brothers said seemed to make a difference to her. "Stop trying to run my life," she protested each time Tricia Ann intervened. But Tricia Ann couldn't resist a big sister's urge to warn Carolyn about the danger of life on the streets. "You're throwing away your life," Tricia Ann told Carolyn repeatedly. "You have so much ahead of you, and you're throwing away your life."

Although Carolyn never seemed to listen, Tricia Ann kept trying. She took her in again and again. She reasoned that if Carolyn had a decent place to live, it would eliminate the need for her to sell her body to buy drugs. Love would heal her baby sister. Instead, Carolyn repaid kindness with thievery. She stole from her family. Then she stole from friends. She stole from neighbors in Clover. When she moved to Gastonia, the big city to Clover residents, she went commercial. She walked into department stores, grabbed merchandise, and ran for the door. She quickly gained the reputation of being a reliable supplier of fine leather coats. "You just asked Carolyn for what you wanted," Tricia Ann says.

But her shoplifting was only one step on the path toward destruction. The money from the clothes and other merchandise she stole paid for her drugs. It was only a matter of time before Carolyn was arrested, handcuffed, and driven away in the backseat of a squad car. Often, when

Gastonia cops busted her for petty crimes, Carolyn stayed in the Gaston County jail for a few weeks sobering up before returning to the streets to begin all over again.

Tricia Ann and John made a regular pilgrimage to the Gaston County courthouse to see Carolyn dressed in orange, looking listless and bored, among the other criminal suspects. Usually she was released with time served. But Tricia Ann and John increasingly worried for their sister. They desperately wanted her to get help. Finally, after ten years of the merry-go-round, instead of asking for mercy, Tricia Ann begged the court to get tough on her sister. "I love my sister, but my sister needs help," she told the judge. "Please get her help because she refuses to get help on her own." The judge was surprised. He was more accustomed to petitions for leniency rather than tough love. He thanked Tricia Ann.

"If we had other family members like you maybe we would stop the drug epidemic," the judge said. He then invited Tricia Ann back to his chambers for a brief conference. He said he understood. He saw the frustration on Tricia Ann's face. When they returned to the courtroom, he seemed composed and ready to mete out his sentence.

"My heart heard your plea for help, and I am going to get her help," he said before sentencing Carolyn to a mandatory six months of residential drug treatment. The judge said that before she could be released, he had to get a report that she was fulfilling her responsibility to get clean. If not, she had to stay another six months.

Tricia Ann sat in the courtroom with her brothers Danny and Spanky; Spanky, like Carolyn, was on the road to criminal ruin. Carolyn wore an orange jumpsuit, her face pale and ashen. She looked unsteady on her feet, as if she needed a fix. She seemed unimpressed and unrepentant. She looked at her sister with flames shooting from her bloodshot eyes. In her drug-affected mind, Carolyn was convinced that if Tricia Ann hadn't requested rehab, the judge would have given her probation and set her free. "I hate you. I hate you. You're not my sister," she yelled as the deputy sheriff led her away. "Get me outta here!"

From the Gaston County jail, Carolyn's next destination was likely the state-run alcohol and drug abuse treatment center located ninety minutes away in Black Mountain, North Carolina.

Carolyn went to a residential detox treatment facility that served drug and alcohol addicts from the thirty-eight most westerly counties in North Carolina. The center would have been perfect for Carolyn. She desperately needed the help, and now she didn't have to pay a red cent for it, because the center operates under the authority of the North Carolina Department of Health and Human Services.

With Carolyn in drug rehab, her siblings relished the brief respite. For a while, at least, Tricia Ann, John, and the others didn't have to worry about the possibility of that late-night phone saying that Carolyn had been found dead of a drug overdose somewhere in an abandoned house or of a bullet from a vengeful drug dealer upset about not getting paid for drugs she had obtained on credit. Ten years after their mother's death, they desperately hoped rehab would help their baby sister make a fresh start. But before she could start over, fate demanded that Carolyn taste the bitter fruit of her sordid past.

A phone call to Tricia Ann finally came. But it wasn't the police or the hospital. It was Carolyn calling from rehab, crying hysterically and inconsolably. Before her admission, the center required Carolyn's social history and a written evaluation of her mental state and her drug problem. Then they formulated a plan of care. Once Carolyn arrived, the staff screened and evaluated her to determine if she needed acute care. They demanded urine and blood samples to ensure that Carolyn hadn't used drugs recently and to test her for sexually transmitted diseases. It would take a few days for all the test results to come back. In the meantime, Carolyn was assigned bed space in the dormitory and a primary therapy counselor. She then underwent orientation.

Counselors employ a certain protocol when a patient tests positive for HIV. The counselor must have visited Carolyn in her dorm and accompanied her to a private room. The two must have sat alone making small talk, with the professional being careful in her choice of words. Carolyn, long skilled at fooling social workers, would have been cagey and deceptive. The counselor would have had the charts that showed her the client's troubled family and personal history. She would have known about Carolyn's fractured relationship with her mother and her life of sex and drugs.

That day in 1989, the counselor would have told Carolyn, in the kindest way possible, "I am sorry to tell you, your test came back positive. You have HIV, which leads to AIDS." The words hit Carolyn like a runaway tire from one of the lumber trucks that rolled through Clover on their way east to the Bowater paper mill in Catawba. Her knees buckled, and the room seemed robbed of air. She fought for breath. She tried to stand, but her legs refused to respond. Carolyn doubled over in her seat and screamed, as if her loud wail would block out the ugly, frightening truth she had just heard.

When the counselor called for orderlies to help Carolyn back to her dorm room, Carolyn's legs refused to carry her. She slumped in bed and stayed there all day. She couldn't eat. She wept constantly.

AIDS wages a battle of attrition on a patient's immune system, leaving her vulnerable to opportunistic infections. Near the end, self-inflicted death, any form of escape, can seem preferable to more pain and suffering. Back in 1989, doctors knew the average person with AIDS could live a fairly healthy and productive life for about seven to ten years, as long as she followed her treatment regimen. Since then, some people, including celebrities like Magic Johnson, have lived with AIDS for more than two decades. But Carolyn couldn't have known that. All she heard was the dreaded word *AIDS*. Being on the wrong end of an HIV diagnosis felt like a death sentence. Carolyn had seen the ashy, scarred skin of friends who contracted AIDS. To her, that fate was worse than having the disease.

Back then, many men and women diagnosed with AIDS saw suicide as the cleanest way to avoid the long, shameful, painful death sentence. People with HIV were seven times more likely to try to end their own lives than uninfected people. Fearing that Carolyn would hurt herself, the staff removed her from the dorm and placed her in a special room where they could monitor her around the clock for three days. "I didn't want to live anymore," Carolyn said years later. "I thought my life was over."

Counselors at the drug treatment center were desperate to pull Carolyn out of her depression, so they suggested that she call her next of kin.

That's when she phoned Tricia Ann screaming as if her hair were on fire. Tricia Ann's husband, Larry, answered the phone and handed it to his wife. "What's wrong?" she asked.

"They say I have the AIDS," Carolyn screamed. "They say I have the AIDS. I am going to die." Tricia Ann heard her sister's words, but it took a minute for them to sink in. The last time she had spoken to Carolyn, she was screaming. Back then Carolyn had directed hate at Tricia Ann; now Carolyn seemed to demand that her sister comfort her, tell her that the tests were wrong, that she was not HIV positive. A staff member took the phone. Tricia Ann wanted to jump in her car and speed the 109 miles to the rehab center and wrap her arms around her baby sister and console her.

Tricia Ann didn't know much about AIDS beyond what she had learned from watching *The Ryan White Story* on ABC television. The movie, which premiered in January 1989, told the story of White, the young Kokomo, Indiana, hemophiliac who contracted AIDS from infected blood during a transfusion. It portrayed his battle with the local school board that tried to keep him out of school. The movie cataloged the fear, ignorance, and bigotry that accompanied much of the early years when the public and the scientific community were still uncertain about how to prevent the spread of HIV and AIDS. The year before, US Surgeon General C. Everett Koop and the CDC mailed a brochure "Understanding AIDS" to every American household. Like most Americans, Tricia Ann must have thought the brochure was junk mail and tossed it into the trash without reading it. All she knew was that AIDS could kill her sister.

After Carolyn hung up the phone, her words kept echoing in Tricia Ann's mind. She couldn't wait to get into her bedroom and lock herself inside her prayer closet. It was the only thing she could do to stop feeling so desperately powerless to help her baby sister.

By 1989, AIDS had been in the public consciousness for eight years. Gay men and intravenous drug users in the big cities were still dying in unprecedented numbers. Carolyn, a black woman living in a small southern town, might have thought herself immune and shielded from HIV. She was dead wrong. But the news wasn't all bad. Two years earlier, the US Food and Drug Administration had approved the first antiretroviral drug, Zidovudine, or AZT, for people with AIDS. AZT was not being touted as a cure, but it could prolong the lives of those infected with the disease. It offered hope of keeping people alive until a cure was found. But hope wasn't cheap. On average AZT prescriptions cost about $10,000 a year.

For decades, health care workers had established methods to slow the spread of sexually transmitted diseases. It required that the infected person volunteer the names of sexual partners and notify them of their possible exposure to infection. Soon after Carolyn's phone call, Larry and Tricia Ann set out to alert Carolyn's boyfriend that he was in danger. They found him at the apartment he had shared with Carolyn in Gastonia, North Carolina. The details of that conversation are etched into Tricia Ann's memory. It is a scene she replays in her mind again and again.

The man sat calmly as Tricia Ann explained the reason for the visit. As she delivered the grim news, he behaved as if she had told him something he already knew, old news. "I'll handle it," he said.

Tricia Ann was taken aback by his lack of emotion. He didn't behave like a man who just learned that his girlfriend might have given him a deadly sexually transmitted disease. He didn't freak out or swear or threaten Carolyn's life as might be expected of a man whose girlfriend might have infected him with HIV/AIDS.

"He handled it too cool," Tricia Ann said. "I always thought she got it from him."

As the couple drove away from the apartment complex, they looked at each other. "He has it," Tricia Ann said to Larry.

"He knew," Larry concurred.

9

PEGRAM BABY

The phone rang with an ominous urgency that signaled bad news. It was late July 1991. A nurse was on the line. Tricia Ann had grown used to these kinds of calls, but it unsettled her nonetheless. The nurse said a woman had been admitted to Gaston Memorial Hospital in labor. Initially, medical staff had no idea who she was because she was unconscious from a drug overdose. For forty-eight hours, doctors had worked feverishly to save the lives of the mother and the baby. "It's your sister, Carolyn Pegram," the nurse told Tricia Ann.

Over the next few weeks, the story emerged of how Carolyn, unconscious and strung out on heroin and crack, had ended up in the emergency room, where she gave birth to a drug-addicted baby boy. There is hardly a stronger bond than between a prospective mother and her unborn fetus. Crack or heroin addiction severs that bond; the ceaseless craving for the next narcotic high is the only thing that matters.

In the months leading up to her due date, as her midsection bulged and shook with the life within her, Carolyn dreamed of having a baby of her own, somebody to love. But that desire paled in comparison to the craving for drugs—crack cocaine or heroin, whatever she could use to fill that syringe and prick her elbow to send that flame of sweetness up her veins and vanquish all her sad thoughts, all the gray and black in her mind, even just for a moment. Carolyn never stopped drinking and drugging throughout her pregnancy. What she ate, her fetus ate; what she drank, her fetus drank; what narcotics she injected into her veins traveled through her bloodstream directly to the body and brain of her developing son. When Carolyn got high, her unborn baby clambered the heights with her; when she crashed, he did likewise, his undeveloped synapses and emotions dragged behind like empty cans attached to the car bumper of newlyweds.

The day Carolyn's water broke, labor pains wracked her body like concentric waves running over a fetid pond. It happened as she shot up at a dealer's house with her dope fiend friends. Carolyn's friends must have panicked initially. After all, they couldn't just pick up the phone and call an ambulance. Theirs was not the kind of address to which they'd want to attract screaming sirens. And what if Carolyn died in the emergency room? Police would return to ask inconvenient questions none of her associates wanted to answer. So with the clarity common to those who live two shades beyond the law, several able-bodied men picked up Carolyn, lugged her to a nearby gas station, dropped her on the ground, and immediately scattered like ants before a garden hose. A few minutes later, an attendant called 911.

As doctors in the ER fought to save the lives of Carolyn and her newborn baby, people in the waiting room at Gaston Memorial must have been glued to the television sets as the cable networks broadcast news that authorities in Indianapolis had arrested World Heavyweight boxing champion Mike Tyson for his alleged rape of Miss Black America contestant Desiree Washington three days earlier. While Carolyn's life hung in the balance, she couldn't tell the doctors her name or what kind of drugs she had ingested. She didn't even know she had become a mother for the first and last time.

After the nurse from Gaston Memorial hung up, Tricia Ann resisted the urge to drop everything and rush to her sister's bedside. She had other priorities, she reasoned. She was tired of neglecting her husband and children for a sister who refused to grow up or take responsibility for her actions. At first her resistance held, but then the phone rang again. It was Aunt Lib, the wife of Tricia Ann's uncle, who worked as a nurse in the Gaston Memorial pediatric care unit. When the EMT crew rushed Carolyn into the emergency room, Aunt Lib had been on vacation. After she returned to work that Wednesday afternoon, she overheard the other nurses talking in hushed tones about the newborn "Pegram baby" who might not survive until the end of the week. Aunt Lib was a Pegram by marriage, and the sound of her family name touched her heart. She soon learned the baby's true identity—and that baby was family. She felt compelled to call Tricia Ann.

As she picked up the receiver, Tricia Ann was surprised to hear Aunt Lib's voice. "Did you know that Carolyn had a baby?" the older woman asked.

"Yes, ma'am," Tricia Ann responded respectfully. No matter that she was married with children of her own, Tricia Ann always reverted to that shy, insecure little girl whenever she spoke to Aunt Lib.

"So why aren't you here taking care of him?" the older woman asked. Tricia Ann struggled to find an answer. She grunted and stumbled, but the words caught in her throat. Before she could speak up, Aunt Lib stepped into the breach. "You can't let that child die with no love," she said. "He's family. He's a Pegram."

Those words struck Tricia Ann's heart like a surgeon's scalpel, and she found herself too weak to resist the wave of emotion that swept over her. So many bad memories were ingrained in that Pegram name, so much tragedy, and so much pain. But this was different. This wasn't an adult receiving just recompense for bad behavior. This was an innocent, the child of her drug-fiend sister, who was also infected with AIDS.

Tricia Ann wept at her aunt's words as if they had accused her and she had been found guilty. When her oldest son, Santo, asked her why she was crying, she replied, "Carolyn's baby is not going to make it."

Her husband was at work, and Tricia Ann felt she couldn't abandon her children. But Santo made her decision easy. "Momma, I want to come," he said. With that they hopped into her car and drove forty minutes to Gaston Memorial and headed straight for the nursery. Inside she washed her hands and donned a hospital gown. Aunt Lib waited at the newborn's incubator.

"Hold him," she told Tricia Ann. "Talk to him. Let him know that somebody loves him, somebody cares." The tiny baby could fit snugly in an adult shoebox. At birth he weighed just twenty-four ounces—a pound and a half. In addition to his drug addiction, the newborn suffered from jaundice. He was irritable from his withdrawal pains, so nurses covered his hands in mittens to prevent him from scratching his face with his sharp fingernails. He breathed with the help of a respirator because his lungs were underdeveloped.

Aunt Lib offered Tricia Ann a rocking chair and then reached into the incubator for the fragile newborn and deposited him in Tricia Ann's waiting arms. She held him and began to talk to him as if his little brain could understand the words she spoke. "I'm your Aunt Trish, and I love you," she told him. "Your momma's name is Carolyn. She loves you, even though she can't say it right now."

As she spoke to the newborn, the fire and brimstone country preacher also begged God for help. "Take him if it's your will, God, but I'd rather if you spared his life. He didn't ask to be born," she prayed. And she prayed some more, then just held him and rocked him in silence for about an hour. She rested briefly, then she rocked him again and pleaded with God some more. When it was time for her to go home, she reluctantly gave the newborn to the nurse in charge. Before she drove home, Tricia Ann walked over to the ICU to visit her sister. But Carolyn remained in no condition to talk.

The next day the phone rang again. It was Aunt Lib calling with news about Carolyn's baby. "You have to come back," she yelled to Tricia Ann. "You can't believe the change in him from yesterday." Overnight the baby's heart rate had strengthened, his breathing had improved, and he clawed less frantically at his face. Aunt Lib wanted Tricia Ann to return and sit with the baby again.

"I sat with him, and I prayed with him again," she says. "I told him to fight."

And fight he did. The baby rallied. Carolyn named him Tremaine and called him Tre. But after all the crack and heroin that had coursed through the infant's blood, it took a while before Tre was out of danger and healthy enough to be discharged from the hospital. July had long turned to August, and Labor Day beckoned by the time he was strong enough to go home. The baby's drug addiction was the least of his problems. He was born to a mother infected with AIDS. That was a big worry for Tricia Ann.

An HIV-infected woman can infect her child during pregnancy, labor, delivery, or breastfeeding. Without proper medical treatment, as many as 30 percent of babies born to women with HIV will become infected. Then and now the vast majority, 90 percent, of those children live in Africa.

At that time in America, prior to the introduction of tried and tested HIV prenatal intervention, about one in four babies born to AIDS-infected mothers became infected. Carolyn's baby could easily have been one of the almost two thousand American babies born with HIV that year. Five years earlier, the CDC had recommended that HIV-positive mothers forgo breastfeeding their babies to reduce the risk of infection. Carolyn was in no shape to breastfeed, so that was not a concern. Antiretroviral therapy during pregnancy, introduced in 1994, would reduce the transmission rate to 2 percent or less, but that was years away.

Would Carolyn's son be HIV positive, meaning that only time separated him from full-blown AIDS? Or would the antibodies in her system provide natural protection for her newborn son? Tricia Ann had no answers, only questions she was deathly afraid to ask. Hospital staff tested the baby for HIV. He initially tested positive. Later, as he grew older, those tests turned negative, and he developed into a healthy little boy.

Meanwhile, Carolyn didn't hang around to mope about her recovering son. She remained at Gaston Memorial for about two weeks before the doctors discharged her.

Deep in her heart, somewhere beneath the addictions and the lies, Carolyn longed to be a good mother. And at first she really tried. After she left the hospital, Carolyn accompanied her sister each day on the trek to the nursery to visit her newborn. As they drove back and forth, she expressed her hopes for the future. She wanted to provide a stable home for her son and see him grow up to graduate from high school—something she and most of her siblings never did.

Tricia Ann listened to her sister. Part of her heart wanted to believe, but the other half was skeptical. She had heard her sister's promises before. She knew that, despite Carolyn's best intentions, her sister was often powerless to resist the urges that stalked her veins. Would motherhood give her the strength?

Tricia Ann didn't have to wait long for the answer. About a week before her nephew's release from the hospital, Tricia Ann noticed her sister's calm demeanor dissolve into a jittery nervousness. Carolyn seemed edgy, as if the old drug cravings, the demons of narcotic desire, had returned. She snapped at her sister. Every little thing upset her.

Then one day, when it was time to visit the hospital, Carolyn remained in bed. She said she wasn't feeling good, so she stayed home. Tricia Ann drove to Gaston Memorial alone. But when she returned to Clover that evening, the house sat empty. The lure of the streets had reclaimed Carolyn. Later that night, as the young woman walked through the front door, Tricia Ann knew immediately that Carolyn was high. Her eyes looked wired. Anger pierced Tricia Ann's heart. She confronted her sister, and she didn't mince words.

"You're high, aren't you?" she asked. Carolyn denied she was on drugs, but her behavior betrayed her. She talked loud and acted hyper, as if she had downed too much coffee. In frustration, Tricia Ann ordered her to bed.

The next morning Tricia Ann told Carolyn that the hospital was ready to let her son come home. A few days later, on Friday morning, Tricia Ann drove to Gastonia, wrapped Tre in a blanket, and brought him home to Clover. They had bought a crib, but since the family was unsure of the baby's fate, they had delayed buying baby clothes and other supplies. So that day, Tricia Ann told her brother John to go buy diapers, formula, bottles, and baby clothes. They stored the baby supplies on the dresser in the room Carolyn shared with her son.

Around 1:30 in the morning, a faint, heartbreaking sound emerged from the bedroom. "The baby is crying," Larry said.

"Carolyn is in there with him," Tricia Ann replied and rolled over and tried to go back to sleep. But the wailing only intensified. Finally, Tricia Ann climbed out of bed and drowsily dragged her feet down the hall to check on the baby boy.

As the light flicked on, all traces of sleep disappeared from Tricia Ann's eyes. The baby lay in the crib sucking on an empty bottle in between his cries. On the other side of the room, Carolyn's bed sat undisturbed, empty, as if no one had slept in it. Carolyn was gone—and so were all the diapers, bottles, clothes, and supplies that had been stacked on the dresser hours before.

"Larry, come in here," Tricia Ann hollered. "She's gone. Look, she done took everything. I don't have Pampers for this baby." Tricia Ann knew right away what had happened. She understood the calculus of drug addiction. Carolyn had stolen the baby's things to sell to buy drugs. Larry fumed. He picked up the phone and reported the theft to the Clover Police Department. He wanted Carolyn arrested. But the police would have to find her first.

When she reappeared three days later, Carolyn nonchalantly walked into the house as if she had just returned from running an errand at the corner store. She behaved as if her disappearance was normal, as if she hadn't abandoned her baby in the middle of the night and stolen his things to buy drugs. But it was a thin façade. She wore the staleness of the unwashed and the same clothes she'd had on when Tricia Ann had last seen her. Her eyes were bloodshot and dilated. Tricia Ann was in no mood to play games.

"You can't stay here," she told her sister. Carolyn looked at Tricia Ann as if she were crazy.

"If I'm leaving, I am going to take my baby," she replied, clearly stoned, speaking loudly as if she were wearing headphones and couldn't hear herself.

"If you go into that room and touch that baby, I'll beat you like a horse," Tricia Ann said.

"I'm going to call the police," Carolyn said.

"I'll get the phone, and I'll call them for you," Tricia Ann said and gave her sister the phone. Minutes after Carolyn dialed 911, a police cruiser pulled into the front yard.

"They are trying to steal my baby," she sobbed as the police officers walked in. The cops tried to calm things. They knew Carolyn and Tricia Ann personally and by reputation. They sympathized with Tricia Ann, but sided with Carolyn. Since it was her baby, Tricia Ann couldn't prevent Carolyn from taking him. That was the last thing Tricia Ann wanted to hear. Her Pegram blood boiled. There was no way, after all the weeks of praying and watching over this baby, she would give him up to this drug fiend, even if that drug fiend were her sister.

"She can't have him, even if it means going to court for a court order," Tricia Ann retorted. "Why don't you test her for drugs? She stole everything the baby had and left the baby screaming and hollering."

Carolyn upped her dramatic performance. "You don't love me," she yelled at her sister. "You just want my baby. You just want to get your hands on the welfare check."

Carolyn walked away empty-handed that day. But that wasn't the only time the police came to the house on Queensgate Road because of Tricia Ann, Carolyn, and Tre. Although the South Carolina Department of Social Services placed the baby in Tricia Ann's care, she didn't gain legal custody of him until much later. While Tre was a toddler, Tricia Ann appeared before a judge to plead that Carolyn shouldn't be allowed to have her son until she kicked her drug habit. They imposed strict rules: Carolyn couldn't see her son alone or take him anywhere. But she tried. One day, when the toddler was about a year old, Carolyn, high on drugs as usual, came by, snuck into her son's bedroom, lifted him out of his crib, and headed for the door before Tricia Ann's sons saw her and sounded the alarm.

"Momma, Carolyn's trying to steal the baby," the children hollered. Tricia Ann caught Carolyn trying to go through the front door with her son under her arm. She had no real destination in her drug-warped mind. Her eyes possessed a craven, desperate look.

"I never wanted to take Tre away from Carolyn. No matter what, she loved her son," Tricia Ann says. "I was hoping one day she would see she had a precious child and she would get her life together for him. I thought if I took custody of him, it would take from her the will to get him back."

But she tried to turn things around. More than anything, Carolyn wanted to be a good mother. She entered drug rehab to prove that she could care adequately for her son.

She tried to put her life back together. She tried to find work. She got clean. And Tricia Ann relented. Carolyn could have her son. She and her son's father moved in together again. Carolyn's life finally seemed straightened out. Her prayers had been answered, Tricia Ann thought. Then the phone rang again.

It was Carolyn's boyfriend. She had returned to the crack pipe. Please come, he pleaded to Tricia Ann. He caught Carolyn trying to steal money out of his wallet to get high, and he jumped on her. She then locked herself in a room and threw the baby out the window as she tried to escape. By the time Tricia Ann arrived at the apartment complex, an ambulance idled out front waiting to take her nephew to be treated for a broken arm. Carolyn had disappeared. Police arrested her boyfriend for child abuse.

Later that day, as Tricia Ann sat at the hospital with the toddler, his arm in a freshly molded cast, Carolyn walked in. She was fidgety and agitated as if wired on drugs. She confessed to throwing the baby out the window. She didn't realize the window was so high above the ground. That episode was the first of a series of incidents in which Carolyn's drug use endangered the life of the baby she so badly wanted to take care of.

After she broke up with her boyfriend, she moved in with a woman friend. Since she had a decent place to live, Tricia Ann asked Carolyn to take custody of her son. She jumped at the chance to be a mother again. But it didn't take long for Carolyn's old habits to erode her maternal instincts. After she left with the boy, Tricia Ann didn't hear from her sister for a few days. That usually meant one of two things, both bad.

Then the phone rang. The caller said he had something Tricia Ann would want—her nephew. A few days earlier, he had sold Carolyn fifty dollars' worth of drugs on credit, and she left the baby as a guarantee she'd return to repay him. But she never came back. Tre still wore the same diaper he was wearing when his mother left him. He stank and his bottom was raw with a rash from sitting in a three-day-old diaper. The drug dealer was desperate to get the baby off his hands. So he promised Tricia Ann that she could come and get the baby if she didn't call the police.

Several days later, after Carolyn learned that Tre was safe at Tricia Ann's, she came around to the house in Clover. But by then Tricia Ann was taking no chances. She had obtained legal custody of her nephew. She also received a restraining order forbidding Carolyn from trying to reclaim the baby she was so ill equipped to care for. The baby would not survive with a mother whose life revolved around getting and staying high. But would his childhood frailties claim him first, or would crime, cocaine, HIV, or heroin claim his delinquent mother?

10

A COMMUNITY
RESPONDS TO AIDS

South Carolina responded belatedly to the epidemic of HIV and AIDS. And much of the state's early response was reactionary, fear-induced legislation meant to placate an ignorant electorate. A South Carolina legislator proposed quarantining those with AIDS. Legislators made it a felony, punishable by up to ten years in prison, for anyone to knowingly infect a partner with HIV. It wasn't until 1990, almost a decade after the advent of AIDS, that Dr. Ball headed a group of health officials, community activists, and people with AIDS to design a statewide plan of HIV testing, treatment, and prevention.

The story of AIDS in a small town sounds like a fatalistic narrative of circumstance and fate intervening to prepare ordinary people to cope with one of life's harshest punishments. It begins and ends with two kinds of people: those for whom tragedy is a catalyst for service and those who use it as an excuse for excess. The history of AIDS in York County, South Carolina, is mostly a narrative of service. Fate placed a person in just the right place more than once. When people stricken with AIDS needed help, these people responded.

The chain of service could begin with any one of several people, but let's start with Rebecca Melton, director of the York County American Red Cross office. Rebecca grew up in Mount Pleasant, South Carolina, a small town outside Charleston. She attended Winthrop University in Rock Hill, a former mill town in search of a new identity. Rebecca always had a heart for helping people. She dreamed of becoming a social worker. One requirement for earning her undergraduate degree was completing an internship with a local social service agency. She chose the American Red Cross.

After she graduated from college in May 1987, Rebecca packed up her belongings and drove home to the Low Country to begin what turned out to be a fruitless job search. Her future lay back in Rock Hill. Later that summer, a supervisor quit in the Red Cross office where Rebecca had worked as an intern. The agency called her. Was she interested in doing the job she had done as an intern?

After a frustrating, jobless summer, of course she was interested. Rebecca repacked her bags and drove back to Rock Hill to work as the director of emergency services for the York County chapter of the American Red Cross, which provided emergency relief to people burned out of their houses or struck by natural disasters.

Rebecca had exactly two years to prepare for the worst natural disaster to face South Carolina in a generation. On September 22, 1989, a month after Rebecca was promoted to director of the York County Red Cross, Hurricane Hugo loomed. The category 5 hurricane leveled the Caribbean islands of Antigua, Montserrat, Guadeloupe, St. Croix, and Puerto Rico en route to a direct hit on South Carolina. Hugo slammed Rebecca's relatives in Mount Pleasant and Charleston and then swept inland toward Rock Hill, where it felled thousands of trees and knocked out the electricity for weeks. More than 180 families needed emergency aid. Homeless families filled the shelters. Months later, Rebecca and her staff still struggled to catch up. But the next major emergency was more subtle, although more frightening.

In the early 1980s, the Red Cross was the major source for replenishing the nation's blood supply. The agency collected about half of the nation's blood donations. But that mission collided head on with the train wreck of the AIDS epidemic. Hemophiliacs, accident victims, and surgery patients relied on donated blood for survival. But blood infected by HIV endangered the lives of those it was supposed to save. Hemophiliacs like tennis great Arthur Ashe and Indiana student Ryan White were victimized by tainted blood donations. Red Cross officials designated the AIDS epidemic as a national emergency. As researchers scrambled to find a reliable test for

HIV to protect the blood supply, Red Cross staff had to improvise. Before anyone could donate blood, employees gave each prospective donor a mini-physical, which included questions about the donor's health and sexual history. They asked a set of questions to determine whether the person had engaged in risky behavior likely to infect the blood supply.

"That was new to our donors," Rebecca said. Those who admitted to using drugs or engaging in gay sex were disqualified immediately. They relied on people to answer truthfully, but donors weren't always honest about their sex lives or their health. "We hoped someone would defer themselves if they thought they would be at risk," Rebecca said. "No one had to know. They could say their blood pressure was high. It was very confidential."

Sometimes the oral screening wasn't enough. She'd get calls from blood donors who said, "I had a letter from the Red Cross saying I should go to my doctor. What should I do?" Rebecca says, "It didn't mean they had HIV, but there was something we picked up in the bloodstream."

Red Cross chapters across the country started providing AIDS education and training. The sessions concentrated on the basics: What are the facts? How do you get it? The training also involved dispelling myths, such as that a person could catch AIDS by simply touching someone with the disease. "We know so much more now," Rebecca says.

The Red Cross also trained instructors to teach others about HIV and AIDS. That training course opened Rebecca's eyes to the harsh stereotypes and gross misinformation in the community. "People thought if I lived in the same house or sat next to them or sat in the same chair I would get AIDS," Rebecca says of the early hysteria. And although many people were anxious to learn more about AIDS, religious conservatism often stood in the way.

"We couldn't say *sex* and could not say people can use a condom," Rebecca said of the rules imposed by some church and civic groups the trainers spoke to. "We would try to explain. We are not teaching against abstinence, just the facts about AIDS."

When Rebecca took the course, one of her classmates was Margaret Jenkins, the tirelessly civic-minded wife of a local high school coaching legend. Soon after the two underwent AIDS training together, Margaret approached Rebecca with a radical proposal.

Margaret Jenkins wore many hats in the Rock Hill community. In addition to being a coach's wife and a mother, she sat on the Red Cross board of directors. She was also the bereavement coordinator for the local hospice agency, Hospice and Community Care. Through her work with the grieving and dying, Margaret discovered that AIDS had come to her hometown. York County hospice's first HIV/AIDS case was an eighty-one-year-old man who contracted AIDS from a blood transfusion.

Margaret joined the newly formed York County AIDS Task Force. Her involvement with the area's fledgling response to AIDS made her aware of the dozens of people who were "grieving their lives." At the time, being HIV positive was a death sentence. A decade into the AIDS epidemic, South Carolina's Department of Health and Environmental Control struggled to mount anything more than a tepid response to the disease. The local county health department staff, lacking resources, reached out to volunteers to start a support group for people with AIDS and HIV, their relatives, and others touched by the disease.

Because of Margaret's experience hosting hospice grief-support groups, it was natural that they called her. But first the group needed a place where people felt safe, where they felt like they belonged—not a church where people could be judgmental. Anyone could attend, no questions asked. There was one requirement: confidentiality.

The Red Cross building, located near the hospital, was perfect. The nature of the agency's business fit nicely. People came and went day and night. Support group members could attend meetings without fear of being "outed" as people with AIDS.

Margaret invited Rebecca to help start the group, thus beginning a five-year partnership. "She was a very compassionate person," Rebecca said. "I thought of myself as the person who could provide the space."

People knew Margaret Jenkins as an energetic, assertive, and persistent woman. Whenever she spoke her mind, which was often, her accent seemed to have migrated from the set of *Gone with the Wind*.

Like many others who are led to social work and missions of mercy, trouble was buried deep in Margaret's DNA. Her version of the family tragedy began with her sixteen-year-old uncle. The scion of a comfortable Savannah family came home one day from football practice and told his mother he felt sick. Before she could put her arms around him, he collapsed and died on the spot. The family summoned Margaret's mother from college in Virginia with news that her brother was ill. When she stepped off the train in Savannah, she learned he was dead. The family fell apart. Divorce followed death. Margaret's grandmother wore black for a year, then lavender the second year, and white for the third year of mourning. Her daughter, Margaret's mother, wore her pain on the inside. She was never quite whole after that tragedy.

"My pain was having a mother who was mentally ill," Margaret says. "She was a manic-depressive in an era when people knew little about the illness." At the time, Margaret says, most people thought the disease was caused by an innate weakness in the person. Doctors and other well-meaning health professionals told manic-depressives to "pull themselves up by their bootstraps." They felt that mentally ill people had control over their sickness.

In a way, the landscape of HIV/AIDS bore a similar message: "You had control of your life. You brought this disease on yourself, if not by sinful behavior at least by your deviant lifestyle. You have no one to blame but yourself."

"Mental illness was a little like AIDS," she says.

Margaret told her story on a midsummer Sunday afternoon in the Rock Hill living room of social worker and educator Linda Ashley. Ever on the move, Margaret had driven down from her mountain condo in western North Carolina just for the occasion. Ashley sat on her right, and Tricia Ann, who had preached a sermon hours earlier, sat on the left, next to the fireplace.

The concept of pain resonated with all three women. Linda Ashley's pain came from her son's suicide in 1989, Tricia Ann's from losing her mother, Annie Mae, to a lifetime of illness and then her family members to AIDS and other maladies. People who have been through great pain recognize it in others.

"They knew that I knew what that pain was," Linda says of her AIDS clients. "They would open up and say things they didn't say to the nurse, they didn't say to the doctor." Each woman had walked on pathways littered with pain. And that pain in some strange way seemed to prepare each of them for an exceptional journey. It gave them the empathy, the strength, the courage, and the willingness to hold the hands of men and women who had made wrong, tragic choices and still love them.

Somehow Margaret turned out all right. From her parents' home in Atlanta she moved to Columbia, where her older sister lived. The University of South Carolina had a reputation for being less of a party school than the University of Georgia in Athens. In Columbia, she met Bob Jenkins, who loved track and football. It marked the start of a lifelong partnership that has lasted for more than half a century.

Bob and Margaret came of age in a South still largely unwilling to acknowledge, much less forsake, its racist legacy. Bob first coached at the Fishburne Military School in Waynesboro, Virginia, a small town nestled at the base of the Blue Ridge Mountains named for Revolutionary War general Anthony Wayne. The couple spent four years in Virginia and in 1961 returned to his home state to coach football and track at the Carlisle Military School in Bamberg County. Bamberg's majority black population had long been dominated by an indifferent white minority, which was bred to believe people of color belonged in a subservient place. Bamberg sat stuck in the mud of rabid racism and anticommunism. The rural community offered fertile soil for groups such as the John Birch Society. During the Cuban Missile Crisis of 1961, as soldiers rode in the backs of trucks down

Highway 301 on their way to active duty in Miami, they passed a full-size billboard that read IMPEACH EARL WARREN. One person waving farewell to the troops said Justice Earl Warren was a flaming "red."

"He was convinced that the Warren Court was a communist organization," Margaret says. Never one to remain silent in the face of bigotry, Margaret spoke up.

"Do you think all the justices are communists?" she asked the protester. His response didn't matter. Right then, Margaret vowed to leave Bamberg as soon as she could. But among the three thousand or so residents of Bamberg, Margaret and Bob met some good people mixed in among the extremists. The place was so small folks knew whether you wore brown or black shoes to church on Sunday.

As the Jenkinses settled into community life, they became friendly with Dr. Michael Watson and his wife, Mary Carolyn. Bob sometimes rode with Dr. Watson's partner, Dr. Dwight Marion, as he made late-night house calls.

As fate would have it, even as Dr. Watson began treating AIDS patients at the county health clinic decades later, Margaret was conducting sessions counseling grieving families, some of whose relatives had died of AIDS.

The Jenkinses left Bamberg in 1965, a historic year in the annals of the South, and headed north to York, the county seat of York County, a place where the KKK could still march with impunity. At York Comprehensive High, Bob was assistant principal, athletic director, and head football and track coach. As the football coach's wife, Margaret knew about community backlash. A two-game losing streak or a loss to an out-of-town rival could prompt hateful late-night phone calls. "If he didn't win, 'the moving van will be in front of the house the next morning,'" the anonymous callers threatened.

Bob Jenkins played the first black player on the York High football team when the school became integrated following the state's decision to opt for school choice instead of all-out desegregation. In 1963, the South Carolina legislature passed a law allowing any student to attend any school where he or she was a minority, no matter where he or she lived. Otherwise schools were segregated. Jim Crow still ruled. Children attended schools in the segregated neighborhoods where they lived. A decade after the historic *Brown v. Board of Education* decision, for the first time a black student could attend a white public school and a white student could attend a black school in South Carolina. It meant that, for the first time in the Palmetto State's history, black students could sit in a classroom alongside their white counterparts. It also meant that for the first time black players could stand shoulder to shoulder with white players on the defensive and offensive lines on the football field. But reactionary forces intervened to delay the inevitable.

In a classic peremptory move, the state high school league ruled that any athlete who did not make a "bona fide residential move" with a parent or guardian was ineligible to play sports for twelve calendar months after a transfer. A dozen black students transferred from York's all-black Jefferson High School to York Comprehensive High in the fall of 1965. Several black students wanted to play football. But because of the rule by the athletic governing body, none could show off his prowess for the Cougars. They had to wait another year before they could wear the team's colors.

"It didn't mean we couldn't coach them," Bob Jenkins says. And that summer, having fulfilled their twelve-month waiting period, they became eligible to play high school football. Four black players showed up on the first day of practice that summer of 1966. And so did a carload of hooded and robed Ku Klux Klansmen. They sat in the stands and watched practice but never uttered a word.

"The first day the kids and coaches asked, 'What should we do?' I said, 'We keep on doing what we've been doing.' They just sat and watched."

The Klansmen must have been impressed, because they returned daily to watch practice for several weeks. But they failed to intimidate either Bob or Margaret. "We knew their pickup truck, we knew their shoes, we knew their hoods, we knew their clothes," she says.

Not long afterward, two prominent boosters from Rock Hill High recruited Bob to coach football and track. Rock Hill was a textile town with pretensions of progress. When Rock Hill built a second high school, Bob moved across town to Northwestern High, where he coached the football team for three seasons.

Meanwhile, the couple embraced life in Rock Hill. High school coaches' wives in small southern towns are usually lonely women robbed of social status by their husband's meager earnings. Margaret managed to escape the pitfalls of poverty and loneliness. While Bob stalked the sidelines on the gridiron and track field, Margaret stayed busy. Like many stay-at-home southern women in her position, she volunteered around the community. She served on the York County Alcohol and Drug Task Force. The guys did most of the talking, while Margaret was the secretary. She took detailed notes, a habit that came in handy as the years passed.

Then fate pushed Margaret in another direction. For years she came home talking about drugs and alcohol and mental illness. Then she turned her focus to death and dying and hospice care after seeing the difference hospice made in the lives of one estranged couple.

Beth, one of her daughters' best friends, was diagnosed with cancer when she was fifteen years old. Before she fell ill, Beth watched her parents undergo an acrimonious divorce. Although Beth's father and mother were bitterly angry at each other, Charlotte Hospice's staff, with skill and patience, brought the couple together for the sake of their dying daughter. They taught the two adults how to focus on what was important in the middle of a tragedy. In so doing, the agency made six years of suffering and dying bearable for that teenager. "Beth died with her two dogs on the bed and her mother and her father holding her hands," Margaret says.

She wanted grieving families in her hometown to have those kinds of options, so she joined a group that was trying to establish a nonprofit hospice service. Some group members had lost a spouse to cancer. Some were clergy. This was more than a decade after Elisabeth Kübler-Ross's groundbreaking work, *On Death and Dying*.

The local hospice started in one room of the Oratory, an autonomous center for Roman Catholic priests in Rock Hill, then moved down the road to the Winthrop University campus before it found a home in a house on the south side of town. Soon afterward, Margaret became the bereavement coordinator. She conducted an eight-week support program for survivors. She visited families. For three years she studied the science of grieving and dying with Kübler-Ross in Virginia.

AIDS changed the way people lived and died. And as the scourge swept across America, from the big cities on the West and East Coasts to every town and hamlet in the Midwest and Deep South, those who cared for the dying struggled to cope with the new reality. Volunteers and nurses at the fledgling community hospice encountered their first AIDS patient in the early 1990s. But staff and volunteers did not readily embrace the call to offer solace to dying AIDS patients. Some early hospice nurses refused to enter rooms with AIDS patients. Others worried that if they treated people with AIDS, other dying people, fearing the stigma, would seek palliative care elsewhere. And if families shunned hospice because of AIDS, the donations would dry up.

Around that time, circumstances gift-wrapped a new mission for Margaret. "People came to me and said, 'Margaret, you have been doing grief work. AIDS patients are grieving their lives.'" It didn't take long for Margaret to step forward. What she saw were mostly gay men who were forced to die without their families' support.

"With AIDS they weren't allowed to grieve in public," she says. But she was also inspired by the courage and honesty of the dying. They usually forgot the pretense and the lies. "They are more real than at any other time in their lives," she says.

By 1990, it was clear to many in the faith community that York County needed to respond to all the death and dying in places hidden far from the headlines. But this was still a very conservative place, where talk about sex, condoms, and homosexuality remained off-limits. Any discussion of same-sex relationships soon devolved into a treatise on Sodom and Gomorrah.

From her work with hospice, Margaret Jenkins and others set out to form one of the earliest support groups for people with HIV and AIDS or family or friends touched by the illness. Margaret and Rebecca worked with the support group for five years. "The nature of the work was difficult," Rebecca says. "People you got close to died."

It was the sort of setting in which people could come and go in relative anonymity. On Wednesday, October 17, 1990, Margaret walked in to convene the first meeting. In attendance were Charles, the son of a well-to-do Rock Hill family; Johnny Plyler, one of the few locals who would admit to being HIV positive on television; navy veteran Chris Blanton, who came to lend support; and Jaime (name changed), a Winthrop co-ed who was HIV positive. She feared her parents finding out more than she feared the disease itself. Jaime had a future she was desperately trying to protect. She was engaged but refused to warn her fiancé about the possible dangers that lurked in their nuptial bed.

After Jaime walked down the aisle, she left town and never returned to the support group. Also at that first meeting were identical twins Larry and Harry, who both contracted HIV from intravenous drug use while they lived in New York, then returned South to live out their last years. Social worker Gerald Weiss spoke to the group about intimacy and sex for people living with a fatal STD.

Charles went to a local mental health center to talk with someone about his condition. No one would see him, and Charles couldn't understand why. And when he tried, he wasn't allowed to have anyone other than family or a guardian accompany him. This event made members of the support group realize that people with HIV and AIDS desperately needed an ombudsman. When Margaret asked Johnny Plyler if he was willing to take on the job, he readily accepted. He went with Charles and answered questions Charles couldn't answer, but they wouldn't allow him into the inner sanctum—the room where the life-and-death, patient-doctor decisions were made. The next meeting, the support group tackled the issue head on. They needed someone to advocate for people with overwhelming physical, medical, and financial needs.

At the time, the state health department in Columbia employed an ombudsman who completed power of attorney forms, living wills, and other documentation for men and women battling life-threatening illnesses. Margaret wrote to the state ombudsman to ask about starting a program in York County. Then she and Johnny drove to Columbia to meet him. He loved the idea of a local AIDS ombudsman, and so the York County area launched a pilot project for the state.

Johnny Plyler was diagnosed with HIV in 1986 and developed AIDS four years later. He believed his personal struggle qualified him to be the first ombudsman, the first official advocate for HIV/AIDS.

Soon after his appointment as the first York County AIDS Ombudsman, Johnny succumbed to his illness. His mother, Dot Plyler, succeeded him to become the second governor-appointed ombudsman. Later, navy veteran Chris Blanton would step forward and give the role a whole new meaning.

11

CHRIS BLANTON

Johnny Plyler dreamed of being an AIDS advocate. His AIDS status gave him credibility, but his illness became a disability. He was willing, but his health prevented him from doing the job.

Chris Blanton was just the opposite. With his tidy moustache, all-American good looks, and southern gentility, Chris could convince any concrete-hearted bureaucrat to do exactly what he wanted. But behind the charm lay much pain born out of a time when his close-knit family was torn apart by divorce and his mother's abandonment.

The Blanton siblings came in a hurry, separated by a year or two at most. Their parents joked that they were doorstep kids. Tammy, the first, arrived in 1965; then a year later came Chris; then a brother just nine months later. A second girl arrived in 1968, the year with the student protests, the marches, the riots, and the looting after the assassination of Dr. Martin Luther King Jr. That was fourteen years after the US Supreme Court had ruled that school segregation was illegal. But the people of South Carolina, like most of the places below the Mason-Dixon line, tried to ignore the decision of liberal judges in Washington. It was not until around 1970 that Rock Hill schools were fully integrated. Back then, the Blanton family—mother and father, two girls, and two boys—lived in a modest ranch house in a working-class, mostly white neighborhood off Cherry Road, the main thoroughfare running north and south through the mill town. Their uncle, who lived next door, also had four kids—fun playmates for the Blanton siblings.

Chris's father, Junior, a welder for a factory in Charlotte, drove thirty miles across the state line to work each day. His mother, Mary, was a pretty, small brunette, who spent her days serving tables at one of Charlotte's many family restaurants.

The Blantons found ways to stay active and happy. On weekends, Junior and the boys fished for carp and catfish in the Catawba River, a waterway that meandered from the North Carolina mountains down to Lake Wateree in South Carolina. The river had lost its verve generations earlier when Duke Energy, the state's dominant utility, dammed the waterway to bring reliable hydroelectric power to the region's textile mills.

On Saturday mornings, when the river was low, Chris and his siblings biked up to the river, rolled their jeans above the knees, and cast their lines from their homemade bamboo fishing rods. Everyone knew that on hot summer days the carp were jumping.

After the July thunderstorms, when the Catawba turned dark and muddy, they'd land eight- and ten-pound catfish on their lines. In the fall, when the leaves turned from green to spectacular orange and the night air was tinged with the aroma of burning oak logs, Chris and his father cleaned their rifles in preparation for deer hunting season.

Chris liked nothing better than to spend the first light of dawn hunting on a Saturday or Sunday morning. As the earth sighed in wisps of white mist, thick enough to hide the deer strolling through the brush, he jammed his rifle against his shoulder, then pressed his index finger against the cold metal trigger until the rifle exploded, the butt recoiled against the meaty portion of his teenage shoulder, and the prey either fell to the ground or scampered away before disappearing into the mist.

Chris didn't play baseball; he didn't even sign up for Pop Warner football. He preferred the solitude of the outdoors, him and nature, his thoughts loud in his head as he and his siblings rambled through the woods out back of his home. And increasingly, since he was thirteen, a seventh-grader at Sullivan Middle, he thought of the secret buried in his heart.

Do you have a girlfriend? A young boy gets little time to dodge the question. As soon as he turns eleven and his voice begins to deepen and lose the high-pitched echo of childhood, adults pepper him with the question. For most boys the question is a dare, a challenge to test the water of love and lust. But for Chris, the question elicited only panic. He had no desire for girls. He enjoyed their company but not in the way other boys did. Fear, rather than desire, consumed him.

What if adults discovered that his heart skipped a beat when he saw some of the boys in the hallway? His worst fear was someone finding out. He knew he was different; the feelings in his heart and the thoughts in his head told him so. His was an experience shared by millions of young boys and girls who felt cursed with an attraction to someone of the same sex. "You don't talk about it to anybody," he says. "You just try to push that to the back of your mind. You just knew."

During adolescence he fought this deep, dark secret, wondering, hoping, praying that it was just a phase he was passing through. Then his internal turmoil was replaced by other worries. The Blanton household dissolved into a battleground as his mother and father quarreled bitterly. The summer he turned fourteen and was anticipating the thrill of freshman year in high school, Chris awoke one day and his mother was gone. Chris was her heart, her pet. He felt as if she had abandoned him. Her floral dresses no longer hung in the clothes closet. He missed her voice around the house. She meant everything to him. Even though he was a teenager, ready to spread his wings, he longed for her affection and approval. He struggled to adjust to her absence.

While Chris struggled to recover from his mother's abandonment, his father didn't sit around moping for long. Soon afterward, a young woman started coming around the house. She was much younger than Chris's mother, perhaps about ten years older than Chris and his siblings. His father's mood changed. He laughed again. He didn't have as much time to fish with Chris and his brother, but at least he seemed happy. A few months after Chris's parents separated, the family packed up and left the house they had inhabited for twelve years. They moved north eight miles to the adjacent town of Fort Mill, a classic textile mill company town dominated by Spring Industries and the Close family.

That September Chris walked into Fort Mill High for the first day of class. The kids were just like his old schoolmates from Rock Hill: children of mill workers mostly, white, gangly descendants of Scotch-Irish settlers of two centuries before. Like their parents, they disliked difference and outsiders. They railed against any behavior that ran contrary to their inherited Presbyterian moral values.

Chris tried to act normal, to be one of the guys. He hunted with his .270 rifle; his fishing rod never gathered dust. During his senior year, he even tried dating a girl. She was a pretty brunette who loved to ride shotgun in the snow white '72 Monte Carlo Chris's father had spray painted with a special mixture from the factory where he worked. For the first time in his life, here was a girl who really made his heart beat fast, who left him at a loss for words. His strong feelings for her surprised and unnerved him. On dates Chris took his new girl to the Putt-Putt miniature golf park in Rock Hill. He took her to the movies, and once even they rode down to the river. They were lying on the hood of his car staring up at the stars that night when two York County sheriff's deputies pulled up and startled them. "Have a pleasant evening," said the deputy behind the wheel before he drove away.

That was Chris's most poignant memory of heterosexual love—no physical contact, no heavy breathing, no stolen kisses, just an intense longing in his heart for this pretty brunette and the maddening confusion in his head over illicit desire he felt powerless to control. Then, as quickly as it started, it ended. There was no formal breakup—just silence and distance. She went back to her old boyfriend. "She broke my heart," he says.

One day almost ten years later, after he came home from the military, after he had come out, the phone rang, and Chris answered. She was surprised that he recognized her voice immediately. How could he forget? She was his only date from high school. She called Chris after she saw his name in the *Rock Hill Herald* newspaper. Out of curiosity, she called to see if it was the same person she had dated those years before. They exchanged pleasantries against a backdrop of awkwardness. Then she was gone.

As his senior year dawned, the confusion in Chris's head wasn't limited to whether he should date a guy or a girl. He had no idea what he wanted to do for a career. He worked at the Bantam Chef restaurant throughout his senior year. His wages paid for gas and spending money. After graduation, he spent many days driving around in his car trying to figure out where he was going. As he drove his Monte Carlo, his radio was silent. There was no soundtrack to his teenage years. He preferred the rustle of the wind in the trees, the silence in a tree stand stalking deer, and the burble of water over the rocks down on the Catawba River to the roar of Friday night football.

Everyone whose counsel he treasured told him to make a decision. But for an unprepared teenager, making a career choice could be the hardest thing in the world. He didn't see himself as college material. At the same time, he didn't enjoy the prospect of slaving in a restaurant for the rest of his life. During that time, he spied a newspaper ad. JOIN THE NAVY, it said. He visited a recruiter, and before long he boarded his first plane flight for Orlando, Florida, heading for basic training.

The Land of Disney felt like landing on the moon compared to Fort Mill, South Carolina. But that was nothing like adjusting to the rigors of navy boot camp. Chris immediately realized he had made a terrible mistake. He hated the navy. He hated the rules, the orders, and the drills. He felt homesick for South Carolina. Chris wished he could just walk up to the drill instructor and announce that he had changed his mind. But he couldn't bring himself to quit. Giving up wasn't in his nature. And what was he going back home to do? Sell burgers and fries?

One day early in basic training, in late summer 1985, a drill instructor put the new recruits through their paces on the sidewalk in front of the barracks. He wanted to see how well the recruits paid attention to orders.

"Turn right! Turn left!" He belted the orders so rapidly the recruits struggled to keep up.

"If you are not facing the right direction, get down and give me fifty!" he yelled.

Chris felt lucky. He was facing the right direction, he thought. All of a sudden, just as loud as he could, the drill instructor screamed in Chris's ear.

"Give me fifty!"

He didn't dare question the drill instructor or he might be ordered to do one hundred pushups. As Chris pushed up and down, he was struck by the realization that someone whom he had just met had complete control over his life. He hated it but was powerless to change it.

"They either make you or break you," he says. "It's not any different from what a prisoner goes through the first couple of months in jail."

His prison analogy seems all the more apt considering the feelings he had kept locked up inside for so long. But if Chris could learn to live with his secrets, he could learn to be a sailor in Uncle Sam's navy. Drill instructors inflicted physical and emotional torture during the daylight hours. Nights brought no relief. At boot camp, recruits slept on bunk beds in dorm-style barracks. Chris occupied the top bunk directly below a vent that blew cold air on him all night. So here was a South Carolina boy in the middle of Florida, cold, homesick, and twisting and turning in his bed at night unable to fall asleep. In desperation, he grabbed an extra blanket to stay warm. The next morning, he hid the blanket under the mattress next to his. That attempt at self-preservation breached military rules. Had it been discovered, the culprit would have been punished with hours of extra pushups, jumping jacks, and running. But somehow it escaped the petty officers' eyes during the unannounced inspections.

"Nobody ever found it."

That hidden blanket, stashed under a mattress, came to symbolize for Chris his secret sexuality, which he managed to hide from the naval brass for the duration of his military career.

As a young, gay military recruit, sidestepping the navy's dragnet was easy enough, Chris found. The delicate matter of sexual orientation arose only when navy counselors asked recruits if they were attracted to people of the same sex. In one session, recruits were shown cartoon characters and asked a series of questions. Once they were inducted into the military, the matter of sexuality didn't come up again unless there was "suspicious behavior." But if anyone was caught actually engaging in homosexual behavior, the navy responded swiftly and without compromise.

Chris saw the navy's zero tolerance policy toward gays up close while he was in boot camp. As part of their training, recruits took two-hour watch duty while everyone else slept. Whenever one particular young sailor stood watch, he tiptoed around the barracks and tucked the sleeping recruits' blankets under their feet. Several times, recruits awoke to find him tucking them in. Eventually the recruits compared stories. A confrontation over the recruit's odd behavior led to questions about his sexuality. He admitted it—he was gay.

It usually took a couple of weeks to get a recruit processed into the navy, but tossing him out was another matter. Naval authorities reacted swiftly. Once outed, the disgraced recruit was barred from mixing with other recruits; he ate alone and slept in separate quarters as if the navy worried that his homosexuality would spread like contagion among the other young men. They didn't even allow the disgraced recruit to pack his own bags. Two MPs removed his personal items from the barracks. One tagged while the other inventoried them. Each time he left his barracks, armed guards escorted him. He ate alone in the mess hall. One day after he finished eating, he stood up and walked down the aisle, passing a long table where Chris and the other recruits sat. Without looking at them, the discharged recruit blurted out, "The cream always rises to the top, and I'm going home first."

Within days he was gone, issued a dishonorable discharge because he had lied to the navy. The incident left Chris shaken. At the same time, it strengthened his resolve to guard the truth about his sexual preference even more fiercely. "It woke me up to the process I would go through if they found out," he says.

At that time, the navy wasn't just trying to weed out gays. They were responding to the threat posed by acquired immune deficiency syndrome. Several months after Chris completed boot camp, the navy introduced testing of all recruits for the HTLV-III virus, which had been linked with AIDS, although a positive test did not necessarily mean that a person would contract the disease. In January 1986, the *Los Angeles Times* reported that seven present and former sailors sued the navy for discharging them because they were HIV positive.

In his eighth week of boot camp, Chris passed the swimming test. Of course he excelled on the firing range; since childhood, guns had been as familiar as household utensils. But just as when he was in high school, Chris struggled to choose where he would serve in the navy. So with one week left in training, he checked the box marked "submarines."

After a week's vacation in Fort Mill, he headed north to Groton, Connecticut, for basic submarine training aboard the USS *Tecumseh*, a James Madison class ballistic missile sub, which was then undergoing repairs. Named for a chief of the Shawnee nation, the *Tecumseh* was a 425-foot-long nuclear-powered sub. It launched in 1964, one hundred years after a Union vessel by the same name was sunk by a Confederate torpedo in the Battle of Mobil Bay. In the early years, the *Tecumseh* and its crew patrolled the Pacific, but after a major overhaul it was reassigned to the Atlantic fleet and based out of Charleston, South Carolina, a few hours drive from Chris's hometown. Chris was among the 130 sailors who served on the two crews, gold and blue, that manned the *Tecumseh*. The blue crew would spend three months aboard the sub while the gold crew was based ashore in the city of North Charleston, and then they would switch. Unlike surface navy vessels, which visited numerous ports of call, the *Tecumseh* only called at San Juan, Puerto Rico, and the Holy Loch submarine base on the Scottish coast. The faces of the men who served aboard the sub can be seen on a website. They look playful, young, fun loving, friendly, and eager.

The cramped quarters aboard the sub took getting used to, especially after the *Tecumseh* emerged from the shipyard with its regular crew and a host of civilians who came along to test the refurbished vessel. With three times as many crew members as beds on board, the men slept in shifts. Three people shared a mattress on the floor in the same cabin. Chris woke up the next person for his shift so he could climb into the bunk.

Submarine crewmen received mail sporadically. When the submarine surfaced or rendezvoused with supply vessels, the crew could dispatch mail, but each letter was, by necessity and security, short. Sailors could only receive mail from those to whom they had given a special form prior to sailing. Letters took up to a month to arrive. Chris soon learned that casual sexual encounters on land never became long-distance relationships while he was away three months at sea.

In peacetime, the submarine sailor must constantly battle his worst enemy, boredom. Aboard the sub, off-duty sailors listened to music on cassette tapes, played cards, read, or watched movies from the *Tecumseh's* well-stocked video library.

Chris chose to work in the torpedo room, where he was one of three sailors rotating on eight-hour shifts. Each shift usually meant sitting for hours killing time or performing routine maintenance, which generally didn't take long. That's when he developed a love for pop music. Thankfully he took his friends' advice to bring along his cassette player. Chris's choice of submarine duty might have been a metaphor for his emotional and sexual life—hidden below the surface, stealthy, quiet, and dangerous. After three months patrolling the Atlantic from the Caribbean to the British Isles, the *Tecumseh's* crew returned home to its North Charleston base.

Aboard a sub, maintaining privacy is hard and keeping secrets harder still. A thousand feet below the surface of the Atlantic, Chris met other gay sailors. Their brief conversations were coded whispers. Submarines are notorious for their sound-carrying ducts and passageways. Gay sailors lived in fear of being overheard discussing their secret lives. In those days, before the introduction of the notorious "Don't ask, don't tell" policy, hundreds of homosexual men and women were summarily discharged from the armed services after their sexual preference was exposed. It seemed Chris's pubescent life of intense secrecy was apt preparation for four years of military service. He learned to keep secrets, to keep his forbidden life-style under wraps.

But if submarine life taught him the discipline of secrecy and duplic-ity, living in Charleston offered the freedom he had longed for since the seventh grade in conservative York County. Back on land, free of the tight confines and rigid military discipline of a nuclear-powered sub, Chris dove headlong into Charleston's gay scene. Several sailors he met aboard the *Tecumseh* introduced him to the Arcade, one of Charleston's best-known gay bars. Charleston is to Presbyterian and Baptist South Carolina what New Orleans is to Roman Catholic Louisiana. The city, with its Civil War–era mansions and cobblestones, is coastal and cosmopolitan, old but mod-ern. Charleston provided a bazaar for Chris to satiate his sexual appetite. The twenty-year-old started venturing out during his off-duty hours. He began meeting other gay men. For the first time in his life he tried to satisfy his need for love as if it were natural, without shame or guilt.

"It opened a whole different world," he says. When he lived in Charles-ton, most of his liaisons were brief; none survived his three-month deploy-ment at sea. Each homecoming meant another search for companionship and sex. "Because you were on the sub three months and three months off, they didn't seem to last," he says. After three months on shore, he returned to sub duty and to being the perfect sailor. He never ran afoul of military regulations. Superiors never wrote him up. His military record was squeaky clean. "You had to learn. It was a coping mechanism; you had to learn to cope," he explains.

Charleston's gay community lived under threat of death. The first AIDS case appeared in 1982. Three years later, by the time Chris disembarked from the *Tecumseh*, AIDS was rampant in the city. Among the close-knit group with whom Chris partied, one guy was HIV positive. To Chris, who had heard the horror stories of gays dying horrible deaths from AIDS, the friend didn't look or act different. He seemed very comfortable with the knowledge he was infected with the virus. Chris and his friends knew the guy was HIV positive, but he didn't talk about it a lot. As close as it was, the issue of AIDS seemed so far away; he felt untouchable, invulnerable, and immune to the dark worm killing gay people in cities throughout America and the rest of the world. All the death, the talk about a plague, seemed distant, like an alternate universe. He indulged his passions, safe sex be damned.

Whenever Chris drove the two and half hours home to Fort Mill, his father and stepmother were always glad to see him. His half-sister was growing fast. He was the same old fun-loving Chris. He was still young enough that his father never pestered him about getting married and settling down. Then, just as suddenly as it had started, his four-year enlistment ended. There never was any question he would re-up.

In 1989 the US military landscape changed. The Berlin Wall fell; the Cold War ended. For the first time in forty years, the world backed away from the precipice of nuclear conflict. Although tensions with China remained high a year after the Tiananmen Square massacre, all indications were that submarine life would remain tedious and unadventurous. Chris loved Charleston, but he longed to return home to his friends and family in Fort Mill. But before he discarded his sailor's uniform for the final time, Chris felt duty bound to handle some unfinished business.

Although he lived openly among Charleston's gay community, he had spent too much time and energy hiding his sexuality from the prying eyes of the US military. He treasured the newfound freedom that civilian life afforded; he didn't want to return home to live in secret. So just before he left the navy, he drove home to talk to his father and stepmother. He had a secret he felt compelled to share.

"I'm gay." Their reaction surprised him. They both smiled and shrugged. They had suspected it for about a year prior to his announcement. "I was really shocked," he recalls. "I thought I had kept the secret better."

A gay family member of his stepmother, Rhonda, had voiced his suspicions that Chris was homosexual. "They had already started thinking about it. They surprised me," he says.

Like a good southern patriarch, his father wasn't very happy about it, but he and his wife were supportive. Chris could move back in with them once he was discharged from the navy. All his uncles, manly men who hunted deer and reveled in the outdoors, just embraced him, recalled Chris's older sister, Tammy. "It took a weight off my shoulders," he says.

But Chris's estranged mother was not nearly as open-minded. Chris had once been her pet, but now she disowned him. When Chris came out, his sister Tammy told their mother. She forbade her son to contact her. "It was almost like finding out that somebody had died," he says.

The last time the two shared the same room was at his maternal grandfather's funeral in 1994. Then his mother introduced his brother and sister to her boss and her husband's boss, but she refused to acknowledge Chris. For a long time he thought about writing a letter to his mother, but then he thought better of it. When he spoke about her, it was more in defiance than in anger at the lingering hurt only a mother could inflict on a wounded son's heart.

"If she doesn't want to speak to me, that's fine," he told himself. "I wasn't going to try to force her to speak to me. It's like having extra bedrooms in your house that are closed up and can't be opened. But I've dealt with it. I've gotten over it."

The navy discharged Chris on a Friday. He gave up his apartment in North Charleston, and by Monday he had packed up his belongings in his burgundy Thunderbird and sped northwest on Interstate 26 on his way home to Fort Mill. Honorable discharge was unaccompanied by a severance. He needed a job. He moved in with his father and stepmother. Soon he was selling oriental rugs for seven dollars an hour plus commission. He was just twenty-five and too young, he thought, to make long-term plans. Friends told him about a gay bar in Rock Hill, but for a while he couldn't find it. When he did, he was unimpressed. It lacked the class of Charleston, but the Charlotte gay bars helped him forget his old haunts near the coast.

Even though he had come out to his family, Chris didn't feel his sexuality was anyone else's business. It wasn't until his boss confronted him that he felt the need to be more open. Back in his hometown, he settled into a quiet, low-key lifestyle. He was never a hardcore partier, although he certainly had a good time in Charleston during his naval service. Now he looked forward to meeting somebody for a long-term relationship, not just for a good time, not just for a one-night stand.

Not long after Chris returned home, his stepmother, being protective of her openly gay stepson in an age of AIDS hysteria, called the health department to ask what services York County was offering. "I was a gay man; I wanted to know what services were offered. By the time I left Charleston there were friends in the group who were HIV positive."

That was when Chris met Margaret Jenkins, who along with Red Cross director Rebecca Melton had formed an HIV/AIDS support group. The sessions were loosely structured and allowed members to voice their concerns. One common theme of the sessions was the frustration people with AIDS had in securing decent medical care, help for their rent and living expenses, and transportation to doctor's appointments and grocery shopping.

Johnny Plyler, one of the most vocal members of the group, talked repeatedly about the need for HIV-positive people to have a representative, someone who understood the government bureaucracy and could advocate on behalf of those applying for disability benefits and other assistance.

Johnny never hid his HIV-positive status. He appeared on the local educational access channel to discuss his illness. He also visited schools. He spoke up at a time when few people would publicly admit they had contracted the virus that causes AIDS.

"We need to do more than just do lunch," Johnny used to tell complacent members of the York County AIDS Task Force, a group initiated by employees at the local county health department in the early 1990s. "I have to live with AIDS every day." Seeing his passion, the York County Task Force leaders offered Johnny the part-time position, but he succumbed to AIDS-related complications before he could take the job.

Chris Blanton wasn't the first choice to become the York County AIDS ombudsman. But to people involved with the support group and those with the illness, he was the best choice. Years earlier he had returned home from the navy determined to find a way to connect with gay life. He had found a sense of community with Margaret Jenkins and the others at the support group. Chris knew whom to talk to and where to go when it came to getting help for the ailing men in the group. His mixture of military formality and southern charm seemed perfect for the job of ombudsman, so the Task Force offered him the position in 1992 after Johnny died. But Chris balked. He couldn't afford to live on seven dollars an hour for ten hours a week. So Johnny's mother took the position and served as ombudsman for six months. Unfortunately, her new part-time income jeopardized her retirement benefits. She too relinquished the job.

Fate and timing forced Chris's hand two years later. In 1994, the owners sold the business where he worked and laid him off. By then the task force was looking for an ombudsman again. Then the task force lobbied the South Carolina governor to specially appoint the ombudsman and endow him or her with the legal authority to act on behalf of people with HIV and AIDS. They offered Chris the job again. By then his financial situation had changed. After he lost his job, he moved back home with his father and stepmother. He could afford to work part-time.

In another part of the country, Chris's soft-spoken manner might have been viewed as a liability. But in the South that could open any door. Chris also possessed the straight posture of a military veteran. He was very respectful. People loved him.

As the ombudsman, he gained access to documents and could deal with home care, crisis intervention, medical referrals, and legal assistance. He could even accompany people with HIV as they met with their physicians inside the consulting room, where the life-and-death decisions were made. He could draft power of attorney papers.

The task force paid Chris to work ten hours a week, but he threw himself into the job—his beeper rang twenty-four hours a day. He never stopped. If clients called at night, Chris responded. He even cooked soup at his place and delivered it to people who were home sick with AIDS. His approach was simple: "Anything going on? Anything I can do to help?"

And he got results. Within the first year, the position expanded from ten to forty hours a week. "He was the ombudsman," Margaret says. "He was no longer Chris with a life."

Most people with AIDS or HIV didn't own a car; they couldn't afford one. And in small rural towns, public transport was scarce or nonexistent. People needed a ride to doctor's appointments, to go grocery shopping, to the support group. The task force had a budget to assist people to pay bills, but it was limited to $150 a month. Chris asked to increase it to $200 a month per client.

Every month, Chris burned through his budget. When he started, the AIDS Task Force had $7,000 in the bank. After the first year, the annual budget jumped to $70,000. While Chris had money to help people with AIDS, not everyone felt comfortable accepting money tainted by the disease.

"We couldn't even put the name of the organization on the check," he says. "We had to put our initials on the check." But even then not all of the grocery stores in the area would accept the check because of the initials—YCATF—York County AIDS Task Force. "They would always ask me what that stood for," he says. If a client shopped at a particular store regularly, Chris would go to the customer service desk and get the check pre-approved to avoid hassles at the cash register.

He served as ombudsman for eight years, from 1994 to 2002. By then the Christopher Clinic, named to honor Chris's years of advocacy, had opened and was caring for the needs of local residents living with AIDS and HIV.

12

ARMED AND DANGEROUS

While Chris Blanton and others in Rock Hill scrambled to make life bearable for the people diagnosed with HIV and AIDS, less than thirty miles west in Clover, Carolyn Pegram, her friends, and some of her siblings spent their days and nights pretending they had never heard of the disease. They could be forgiven for wanting to forget. The decade after Annie Mae's death was unkind to her children. Drug use, criminal activity, and tragedy marked those years. Siblings raised in a household where they were taught to fear God lived by their own rules.

It started with William, who was shot and wounded even as his mother lay dying in May 1979. Then there was Spanky, nicknamed after the *Little Rascals* character; Spanky had a relatively comfortable upbringing. After his mother fell ill, an aunt took him in and treated Spanky like her favorite son. She bought him nice clothes. She pampered and petted him. But the indulgence backfired. Rather than prepare him for a tough life ahead, it spoiled him. He took to the streets. He dabbled in drugs.

First it was marijuana, and then crack cocaine, the destroyer of dreams. And crack habits are jealous—they demand an addict's undivided loyalty. The demands of an insatiable drug craving drove Spanky to burglary. He broke into houses and sold stolen merchandise for drug money. His passion became his avocation. All of his proceeds disappeared in a smokey haze of crack cocaine. Even as Carolyn ran the streets in the days of 1991, her older brother had embarked on a one-man crime wave. North Carolina Department of Corrections records show that Spanky stole property worth over

$200 on December 31, 1990. That was a misdemeanor for which he was given a suspended sentence and probation on April 8, 1991.

But the Gaston County prosecutor and judge could not have known that, even as they gave Spanky a lecture and his freedom, he was engaged in a massive burglary spree to pay for his drug habit. His North Carolina Department of Correction online file spells out Spanky's itinerary of burglary. More than twenty break-ins occurred in the nine-month period from December 1990 to September 1991:

December 23, 1990: larceny.

February 20, 1990: theft of property of over $1,000, a class H felony.

March 15, 1990: stole over $1,000 worth of property from his employer.

Those crimes surfaced after he was arrested. Tricia Ann said later that after Spanky was arrested, he drove around Gaston County with detectives pointing out all the properties he had broken into.

In July 1991, while Carolyn lay comatose in a hospital bed and as Tricia Ann prayed for God to spare the baby's life, Spanky burglarized properties. The day before Carolyn gave birth to her baby, her brother broke into a house in another section of Gaston County. During an eighteen-day binge, from August 25 to September 12, 1991, Spanky committed seventeen incidents of breaking and entering, records show.

Tricia Ann recalls that after Spanky was arrested that September, he confessed to everything. Justice was unusually swift. On October 11, 1991, less than a month after he committed his last break-in, Spanky was convicted of about forty counts of burglary, larceny, and breaking and entering. The judge sentenced him to life in prison. At the time he was not yet twenty-seven years old.

The day Spanky was to be sentenced, Tricia Ann temporarily set aside caring for her young nephew so she could attend the court proceedings. Tears filled her eyes as Gaston County sheriff's deputies led her brother off in shackles en route to Central Prison in Raleigh, North Carolina. But Tricia Ann couldn't spend too much energy mourning for her brother. He should have known better; more important, a newborn baby still needed her care and attention. By then, the initial excitement of motherhood had worn off for Carolyn and she had returned to wandering on the streets.

Spanky's life sentence proved to be no deterrent for his baby sister. She resumed her pursuit of a daily drug fix with passion in an almost suicidal attempt to still the disquiet in her mind. "I was doing drugs every day, all day long," she told me one day in 2000. The pain and disappointment of a life wasted and poorly lived created an ever-deepening void she felt compelled to fill. But even if drugs couldn't fill the emptiness, the narcotic high helped Carolyn forget, if only briefly, the death sentence coursing through her veins. She tried to forget she had HIV. Even though she hadn't begun to get sick, in Carolyn's mind there was no difference between testing positive for the virus and having full-blown AIDS.

"So many times I laid down with the intention of not waking up," she said. As her desire for drugs increased and her resistance spiraled, Carolyn risked more and more to get money to pay for her habit. She would get high or die trying. Her business model relied on shoplifting excursions to the mall. Her friends in Clover knew where to go when they wanted a new outfit or a leather jacket for a night on the town. Carolyn could deliver the items promptly. She would stroll into Belk's or some other department store, snatch clothes, and run for the door. She even delivered clothes with the anti-shoplifting tags still attached.

On October 11, 1992, a year after her brother was sentenced for his life of crime, Carolyn was forced to test her luck in the courtroom. Cops had arrested her for shoplifting, a misdemeanor for which she was given probation and a suspended sentence. Whatever lesson the judge wanted to teach her, it was lost on Carolyn's drug-fogged brain. Within weeks, she returned to the streets. She had the same old habits but a new level of desperation.

As all fifty states celebrated the Martin Luther King Jr. holiday for the first time on Monday, January 18, 1993, stores hyped sales to attract bargain hunters. To Carolyn, the hordes of shoppers were merely potential victims; their casual attitude and loaded shopping bags made them easy prey. As two white women, a mother and daughter, headed for Target to return some of the younger woman's wedding gifts, Carolyn grabbed the gifts and their pocketbooks and fled in a car toward the state line. Several hours later, Tricia Ann was at home taking it easy on her day off when she heard a rustling noise outside the back bedroom window. Out of curiosity, she poked her head out the window only to find a law enforcement officer with a rifle pointing in her face. She jumped back in shock as she saw the show of force in her backyard. The officers were looking for Carolyn. Her sister was a wanted woman. She was being sought for common law robbery, a felony, and attempted robbery. Investigators recovered the pocketbook of one of the victims sitting on the seat of Carolyn's getaway car.

Tricia Ann loved her sister, but she hoped and prayed that a judge would send Carolyn to prison—finally. If her sister were locked up, she reasoned, then Carolyn would get help to cure her drug addiction; she would get treatment for her HIV. After all those years of running and drugging, her body could not resist the deadly virus much longer. Prison might just save and extend Carolyn's life.

Carolyn was convicted on May 11, 1993. But Tricia Ann didn't get her wish. A lenient judge sentenced Carolyn to a maximum of nine years in prison. But instead of sending her straight to prison, the judge gave her probation and a suspended sentence. She would spend another two years on the street before her luck ran out and she would finally see the inside of a state penitentiary.

Research shows that many women who end up in state prison suffer from drug or alcohol addiction. Their crimes are usually nonviolent, desperate attempts to get money to pay for drugs. Many are sent to prison after being nabbed in a random drug test. Miraculously, Carolyn stayed out of prison for the first two years of her probation.

Soon after New Year's Day 1995, Carolyn visited her probation officer and failed her drug test. After years of gaming the system, she got caught. Perhaps it was a cry for help. After all, she would have been much too proud, much too stubborn, to simply admit her addiction and her inability to break free from drugs and the fast life.

The state revoked her probation on January 30, 1995, and a week later Carolyn rode four hours by bus to the North Carolina Correctional

Institution for Women in Raleigh, the entry point into the state prison system for all female convicted felons. During that first week, Carolyn would have undergone a battery of tests to check her medical and mental state as well as to ascertain her dependence on drugs and alcohol. At that time, whenever a prisoner entered prison, staff relied on the new inmate to disclose any illnesses, including HIV or AIDS. Given Carolyn's callous nature, she kept quiet. Inmates with AIDS were picked on, shunned, and despised. Even without mandatory testing, that year's records show 521 of Carolyn's fellow North Carolina inmates tested HIV positive.

In prison, inmates earn privileges with good behavior. Typically women who break the rules at minimum-security prisons are sent back to NC Correctional Institute for Women in Raleigh. Inmates must either earn their way or be close to release to get sent to a place like Fountain Correctional Center for Women, a minimum-security prison in Rocky Mount, in the far northeast of the state, along the infamous poverty-stricken I-95 corridor. Carolyn was convincing. Several weeks after she reached Raleigh, she boarded a bus with inmates heading to Fountain.

The 583-bed prison was the first prison for women in the state to participate in the community work program, which allowed inmates to perform various short-term, manual labor jobs for local governments. Two crews from Fountain landscaped and painted. In May 1995, not long after Carolyn arrived, about a dozen Fountain inmates drove to Wilson to do clerical, kitchen, laundry, and housekeeping jobs in a nursing home. Carolyn worked as a janitor on the twenty-five-acre prison campus.

Typically, the well-behaved inmates get the plum work assignments—outside the prison walls. Carolyn was no model inmate. North Carolina Department of Corrections records show that on April 18, 1995, she was punished for using profane language. A day later she was punished again for possessing nonthreatening contraband. Five weeks later, on May 26, 1995, as she struggled to adjust to the rigors of prison life after over a decade of license on the streets, Carolyn was disciplined again, for disobeying orders. The records show no details of what happened, but it is easy to picture the petulant, rebellious Carolyn chafing against the regulations and trying to bend and skirt the rules at every turn. Whatever her punishment, it failed as a deterrent. Then nature intervened.

The human immunodeficiency virus damages a person's body by destroying CD4+ T cells, which are essential to helping the body thwart disease. Within several months of contracting HIV, some people exhibit flu-like symptoms that linger for a week or two, while some show no symptoms at all. Some people, like Carolyn, may feel and look healthy for years even without treatment or regular doctor visits. Untreated, early HIV infection is often associated with cardiovascular disease, kidney disease, liver disease, and cancer. Until she arrived in prison, Carolyn had been untroubled by any of those maladies. She had spent six years in drug-induced denial. However, even if she felt healthy, HIV coursed through her body. With her drug abuse, poor eating habits, and sleepless days and nights, there was no telling how much collateral damage the virus had wreaked on her still voluptuous body. She couldn't pretend forever. In February 1996, prison records show, the years of neglect and denial finally overtook her. Carolyn developed a cough and a fever, which soon worsened. She struggled to breathe. She contracted pneumonia. During the early years of the AIDS outbreak, any time someone fell sick with what was then called *Pneumocystis carinii* pneumonia (PCP), doctors would begin speculating about whether the patient had AIDS. PCP is considered an AIDS-defining illness because it is rare in individuals with healthy immune systems. But PCP had become the most common of the opportunistic diseases that laid low people with AIDS. Originally researchers thought PCP was caused by a one-celled organism called *Pneumocystis carinii*, but later research showed the pneumonia was caused by a fungus, *Pneumocystis jiroveci*.

When she fell ill and her condition worsened, prison doctors transferred Carolyn from the Rocky Mount prison to the larger Women's Correctional Institute in Raleigh. The previous year, more than forty-five hundred inmates had died of AIDS in federal and state prisons. Prison doctors worried that Carolyn might be added to those grim statistics. Since the prison did not have the staff or the know-how to treat Carolyn's advanced condition, an ambulance transported her to a community hospital. For several weeks her life hung in the balance. She lay almost comatose, breathing with the help of a ventilator.

When the phone rang at Queensgate Road in February 1996, the news sounded grave. Prison officials summoned Tricia Ann and her siblings to pay their last respects. "I almost died," Carolyn told me later. "The prison told my family I wasn't going to make it." Although Carolyn was barely conscious, she wasn't just worried about survival. She didn't mind being in prison, but she didn't want to die there. She sobbed and wept, as if shame was a whole new encounter. Somewhere, somehow, the rebel who had survived life on the drug-infested streets of Clover and Gastonia found the strength to fight. Maybe Annie Mae's prayers were finally being answered. With the help of antiretroviral drugs, after three weeks she walked out of the hospital and headed back to Fountain prison.

Coincidentally, Carolyn's arrival in the North Carolina state prison system occurred at a time when corrections officials were finally taking an aggressive stand to slow the spread of AIDS among inmates. In April 1995, soon after Carolyn walked into Fountain, the state hired a dozen nurse clinicians and assigned one to each of the state prison intake centers to provide one-on-one care for inmates who had tested positive for HIV or AIDS. At that time, testing was still voluntary. Even if an inmate had the symptoms for AIDS, she could still live in denial.

Carolyn's HIV status went unnoticed until she ended up in the hospital. Once she was released from the hospital and returned to Fountain, a nurse contacted her immediately and began to counsel her. The nurse supervised Carolyn's medication. She educated her about her illness. And for the first time, Carolyn willingly began to take her AIDS meds. Her timing couldn't have been better. Bowing to pressure from AIDS activists, the US Food and Drug Administration approved the first protease inhibitor, Saquinavir, in record time. It signaled the start of a hopeful new era of highly active antiretroviral therapy that would increase the longevity of people living with HIV and AIDS. The Centers for Disease Control reported that between 1995 and 2006, the number of state inmates who died from AIDS-related causes decreased 85 percent, from 1,010 to 155.

That decline was due primarily to better prison health care and more effective medicines.

That near miss might have prompted most inmates to change their behavior. For Carolyn it did only briefly. On May 22, 1996, three months after her release from the hospital, she disobeyed orders and was written up for the first time in almost a year. She must have hit a bad patch around the anniversary of her mother's death, because Carolyn was in trouble again a week later on May 29. Her rebellion died hard. Three days before Christmas 1996, she disobeyed orders and was again punished. The records show that her final infractions—disobeying orders and using profanity— happened on the same day, on February 22, 1997, near her two-year anniversary behind bars.

Surviving a near-death illness gave Carolyn renewed vigor. She wanted to live for her son. A Polaroid picture of Carolyn shows her sitting next to her son during one of his rare visits to see her in prison. He is six or seven. She is dressed in long skirt, T-shirt, white socks, and sneakers. The high cheekbones bequeathed to her by Annie Mae shine from her face, like Palmetto peaches waiting to be picked.

While in prison, Carolyn came home twice, but each time her homecoming was mournful. Her older brother Woody died on April 6, 1997. And her father, Samuel Pegram, the man who used to joke, "Bury me standing up," died of cancer three weeks later on April 30, 1997. Carolyn hated him. He was gone by the time she was old enough to know him. Still, it was an excuse to come home, and she did. Tricia Ann wept for her father, but Carolyn didn't. She was beyond tears. Carolyn was never one to pretend. But that homecoming was a precursor to her freedom.

The absence of serious jail infractions in the latter stages of her prison term worked in Carolyn's favor. North Carolina inmates convicted before structured sentencing was introduced in 1994 could rapidly knock time off their prison terms. Good conduct credit automatically reduced sentences by one day for every day inmates serve with good behavior and without an infraction. Inmates also received credit for participating in work or program activities and doing overtime. Carolyn worked as a janitor. When she was first convicted in 1993, Carolyn was sentenced to nine years in prison and spent the first two years out on probation. After she violated her probation and entered prison in 1995, her projected release date was January 29, 1999. She walked out of Fountain a free woman on July 17, 1997, eighteen months early. But when she returned home from prison, AIDS had already begun to claim some of Carolyn's old friends and neighbors.

13

CLIFF

The life and death of Clifton "Cliff" Caldwell best exemplified the story of AIDS in Clover.

It was business as usual in Alexander's Barber Shop in 1995. Cliff stood over a man's head. He was tall and slim. His face resembled a younger Bill Cosby, but he had the skinny frame of a New Edition Bobby Brown. Mervin Alexander, the owner, stood at his usual spot with his clippers and scissors. Alexander's Barber Shop and Quick Stop is a one-story brick-faced building with a burgundy aluminum roof and a covered open porch that sits on the corner of Marietta and Kings Mountain Streets. The barbershop sits a mere four hundred yards from Clover Community Cemetery, the black burial ground.

Alexander's was more than a place where people came to get their hair cut. It was a communal place. Alexander, a Vietnam veteran, worked at that location before he bought the place and changed the name in the late 1970s. Locals liked to gather in the shop to hear Cliff's recounting of his trips and adventures. He lived out loud. Cruises, shopping trips, carnivals—his life was one long excursion. Standing on his feet cutting hair Tuesdays through Saturdays was merely the price he paid for his good life.

Cliff was always neatly dressed, his dreadlocks tidily done. They fell down to his shoulders. That day he was entertaining as usual as he hop-scotched from one subject to the next. But as he spoke, one of his long dreadlocks slipped from his head and fell to the floor.

In a barbershop, hair routinely falls to the floor unnoticed and without comment. It is the nature of the business. But when hair falls to the ground without the aid of scissors or blade, and when that hair belongs to the barber, not the customer, the patrons will notice. And that day in Alexander's, as Cliff's dreadlocks fell out like a patient losing his hair from chemotherapy, they sure did notice. One occupant asked the question that was on the tip of everyone's tongue.

"Cliff, why are your dreads falling out?" Cliff always had a quick reply for every question, but for once he was stumped. Words failed him. His countenance fell; his mood changed. He was quiet for the rest of the day. After Mervin Alexander closed up the barbershop at the end of business, Cliff packed his tools into his bag. As he did, there must have been an air of finality about his movements, the methodical manner of a man who knew his days at work and in life were surely numbered. That day Cliff went home to his apartment, packed his things, and left town. He never showed his face in Clover again.

Cliff was born on March 10, 1958. He came from a typically large southern family—six sisters and five brothers. At some point, Cliff's father packed up and, like many southern men, headed for New York City.

His old friend Doris remembers that from an early age Cliff was good with hair. He was meticulous. The two met at Clover High School. And although Doris was about three years older, the two found kinship. There was just something about Cliff. He was fun.

Doris knew Cliff was gay from the start. He never tried to hide it, although he didn't flaunt his sexuality the way some of his friends did. In Cloverdale, it wouldn't have mattered. In many small towns, men are fearful about being known as gay, but in the Cloverdale neighborhood there was a certain acceptance. Flamboyant gay men were accepted if not celebrated. Just about everyone had a friend or relative who turned out that way.

Cliff graduated from Clover High in 1976. That fall he enrolled in Livingstone College, a historically black school in Salisbury, North Carolina, founded by the African Methodist Episcopal Zion Church. But he only attended Livingstone for one semester before he dropped out. Like many young black men in the South, Cliff was sidetracked for a while. Then, like his boss, Alexander, Cliff enrolled at Denmark Technical College to learn about hair. Denmark sits about 150 miles south of Clover, a stone's throw from where Dr. Mike Watson was practicing medicine at the time. Cliff must have felt at home in Denmark—at the time the town of about two thousand people was 85 percent black.

Although he always dabbled in hair, South Carolina state records show he didn't secure his barber's license until June 23, 1986. When he returned to Clover with his barber certificate, he took over a chair at Alexander's.

He was good. Although he mainly cut men's hair, the women loved his touch. But none like Doris. He permed, washed, and styled her hair. But no matter how close they were, she always had to pay him. "He'd always say, 'I don't mix business and friendship.'"

Cliff could also be vengeful if you crossed him. At one point, Doris stopped going to Cliff to do her hair and defected to a stylist in Rock Hill. Before one of their trips to Jamaica, Doris didn't make it to the hairdresser. So there she was getting ready to fly to Jamaica in style with her hair undone. In desperation, she asked Cliff. He politely refused. Professional pride, he called it. She had dumped him for another hairstylist, so he felt like a spurned lover.

That minor disagreement aside, the two were inseparable for much of the 1980s and early '90s. They flew to Ocho Rios, Jamaica, on vacation. They drove to New York City to shop. They drove west to New Orleans for Mardi Gras. They drove south to Fort Lauderdale. Each time they arrived in South Florida, Doris checked into a motel room while Cliff stayed at his boyfriend's home. Doris never pried. The reunited lovers would come and pick up Doris, and the trio partied together.

Cliff especially reveled in seducing the macho men. It gave him a sense of power. Whenever he passed them on the street and they ignored his greetings, he didn't hesitate to embarrass them on the spot. He didn't allow the down low guys, those who acted straight in the daylight but covertly enjoyed gay sex, to disrespect him.

Cliff was a fun companion and he provided protection. Men didn't hit on Doris as much if Cliff was around. Plus, she loved the way he eyed the men to whom he was attracted. He flirted as much with the men as she allowed herself to. The first time Doris entered a gay bar, Cliff took her. Once he took her to Scorpio's lounge in Charlotte, an interracial gay bar, where doctors, lawyers, bankers, and the cream of the city's gay life partied. For years, the two were inseparable on the nightclub scene. At some point, though, the two grew apart, Doris remembers. Doris began dating a man who was both jealous of Doris's friendship with Cliff and uncomfortable being around gay men. "We would be together but not hanging out like we used to," she recalls.

Cliff was Orlando Tate's barber from early 1994 until Cliff dropped out of sight a year and a half later. He cut Orlando's hair about once a month. A decade younger than Cliff, Orlando admired the barber's style and talent. Cliff sang and danced. He also helped found the Clover Mass Choir, a nondenominational group of singers from Clover and York that evolved into what is now called the Clover Community Choir.

When Orlando sat in Cliff's chair for a haircut, he looked forward to his barber's take on topical issues. The plight of the black man was always on Cliff's mind. "Whenever I talked to Cliff, we had real conversations—man to man," Orlando says. He valued Cliff's opinion. At the time, Orlando had just moved back to Clover to teach and coach. Cliff was always encouraging. "Keep doing what you're doing," Cliff told him. "Don't have a one-track mind. Do all the things you want to do in life. See the world."

As the two men spoke, Orlando began to suspect Cliff's health was failing. His barber dropped hints. "My health isn't what it used to be," Cliff said. Then Cliff began to wear a scarf around his neck even on hot summer days. Neighbors whispered that he was trying to cover the lesions on his neck. When Cliff disappeared from Clover, he left without a word to Doris, who by then had moved across the state line to Gastonia, North Carolina. Then she heard the rumors.

She finally drove to Rock Hill to see him in Piedmont Medical Center not long before he died. Doris was devastated by his appearance.

"Why couldn't you tell me?" she asked. He seemed to have aged fifteen years. If Cliff was slim before, now he seemed downright skinny. He moved slower. "I could have come to pick you up," Doris told him. But even though he was thinner and paler than before, some things hadn't changed. "He was still just Cliff," Doris says.

That was the last time Doris saw him alive. Friends called her about a week later with the news. Cliff died at the home of his aunt on May 11, 1996. He was forty-eight. On June 3, 1996, three weeks after Cliff's death, his state barber's license expired.

For Doris, Cliff's death was a double loss. She lost a friend and a companion. It was also a reminder that AIDS was stealing people she loved and she was powerless to protect them. Talking about Cliff more than fifteen years later, she couldn't help but remember her younger brother, Maury, who also died of AIDS. Because Maury seemed cursed to steal, he spent more of his short life in prison than being free. Even as a young boy, whenever Maury accompanied his mother to the store he would steal something.

"He'd say he wasn't stealing; he was borrowing," Doris says. A judge sentenced Maury to reform school when he was ten years old. After that his life was made of brief intervals of freedom separated by long spells behind bars.

Maury was the same age as Carolyn. They ran around together. They pillaged the same stores. She stole leather coats and clothes. He stole clothes and jewelry. And, of course, perfume. Maury was obsessed with the fragrance of colognes and perfumes. Tricia Ann remembers he came by and sold her some Navy perfume for five dollars.

But Maury was intelligent. He was talented. He could draw and paint as if he were a professional artist. After he served time in juvenile hall, he came back to graduate with his Clover High School class. But Maury was also a drug addict. His shoplifting paid for his addiction. He was among those who returned from prison looking thin as a pine needle. He had contracted AIDS from his years of drug use. He frequented the house near Roosevelt Park, the one they called "the hill," where the local druggies congregated to shoot up heroin and exchange needles.

One by one, those men and women withered and died of AIDS. Maury's turn was approaching. One day, near the end, Maury went to the drugstore to get his medicine. While his mother waited for him outside in the car, a police officer pulled up, arrested Maury, and drove him to the local lockup. Doris's mother came to collect her so they could visit Maury. It seemed as if they had spent more time looking at Maury through cell bars. "Momma took him to get his medicine, and he was trying to steal. They booked him and let him go," Doris explains.

By then Maury was much too ill to withstand the rigors of prison life. Near the end, Maury tried his best to change. He started going to a white evangelical church in Clover. He wrote letters to God. He lived at home with his mother, and nurses came daily to bathe him and feed him. In the final months, Doris drove Maury to Myrtle Beach. But Maury was tired of living. He couldn't help himself. He hated being an invalid. He gave up. He was in his thirties when he died.

For Doris and her neighbors in Clover, losing a sibling to AIDS hurt. But it was nothing like the fear and panic that gripped the streets of Cloverdale after Cliff died. So many of the people with whom Doris grew up were caught in the snare of shared needles and careless sex. "They all infected each other. They go from one person to the next to the next," Doris says. "That group was just the tip of the iceberg."

Soon after Cliff died, word spread in Cloverdale about a list with the names of forty-eight people with whom he had had sex. It usually takes several years before the infection, if untreated, blossoms into AIDS. Too many people preferred not to know if they had been infected. "Some people refused to take the call; others just didn't get tested," Tricia Ann says. She knew of at least three people on the list who tested HIV positive and later died.

One of the names on the list was Robert "Robbie" Hall, another local barber, who like Cliff had trained at Denmark Technical. When people heard he was on Cliff's list, he lost clients. Robbie left town and headed for Charleston, where his talents mattered more than his sexual preference.

Within weeks of Cliff's death, Linda Ashley was hired as a case manager. Her job was to find those Clover residents who were HIV positive and convince them to get help. But first Linda had to grasp the cultural nuances of black, white, and being HIV positive in a small place like Clover.

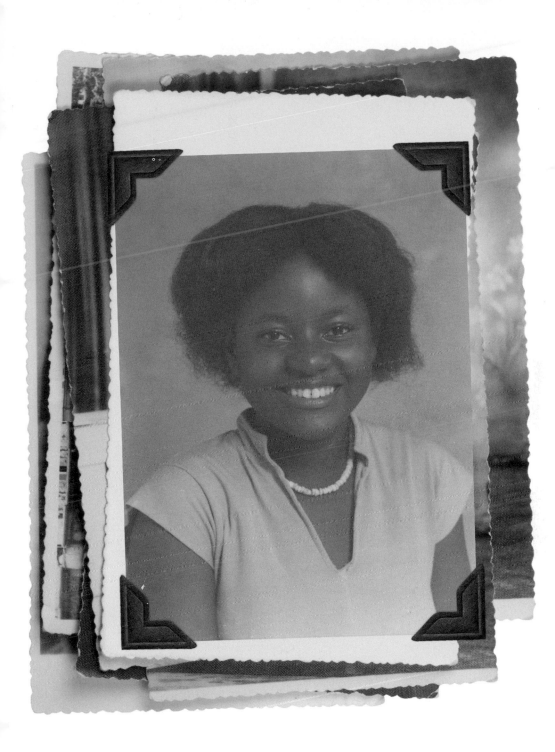

Happier times: Carolyn Pegram in the fifth or sixth grade.

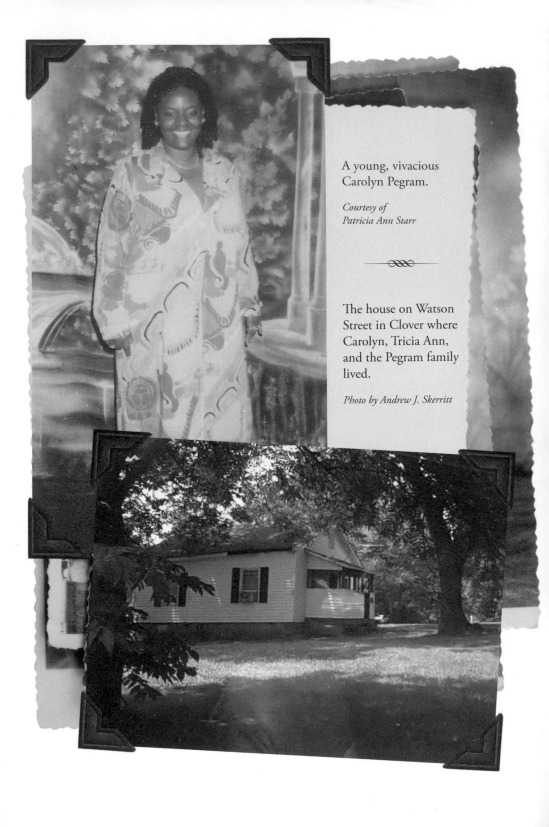

A young, vivacious Carolyn Pegram.

Courtesy of Patricia Ann Starr

The house on Watson Street in Clover where Carolyn, Tricia Ann, and the Pegram family lived.

Photo by Andrew J. Skerritt

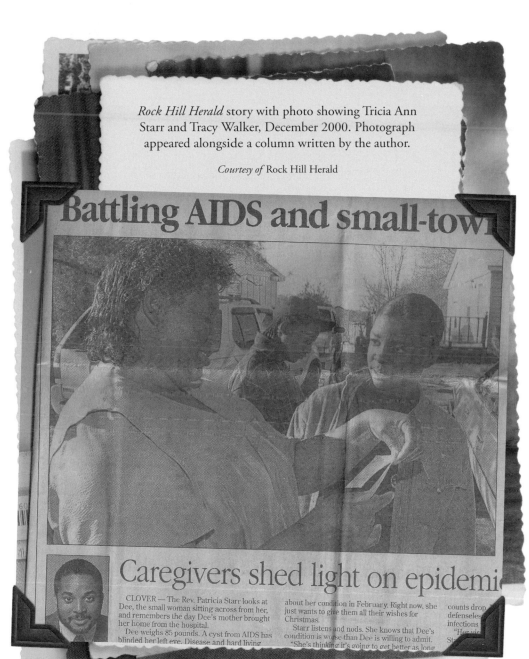

Rock Hill Herald story with photo showing Tricia Ann Starr and Tracy Walker, December 2000. Photograph appeared alongside a column written by the author.

Courtesy of Rock Hill Herald

Battling AIDS and small-tow[n]

Caregivers shed light on epidemi[c]

CLOVER — The Rev. Patricia Starr looks at Dee, the small woman sitting across from her, and remembers the day Dee's mother brought her home from the hospital.

Dee weighs 85 pounds. A cyst from AIDS has blinded her left eye. Disease and hard living

about her condition in February. Right now, she just wants to give them all their wishes for Christmas.

Starr listens and nods. She knows that Dee's condition is worse than Dee is willing to admit.

"She's thinking it's going to get better as long

counts drop defenseles[s] infections

"Her vi[...]

St[...]

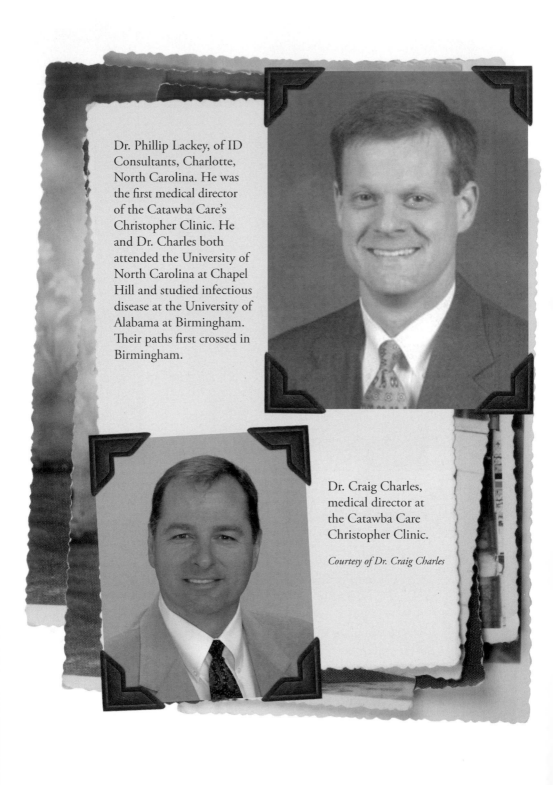

Dr. Phillip Lackey, of ID Consultants, Charlotte, North Carolina. He was the first medical director of the Catawba Care's Christopher Clinic. He and Dr. Charles both attended the University of North Carolina at Chapel Hill and studied infectious disease at the University of Alabama at Birmingham. Their paths first crossed in Birmingham.

Dr. Craig Charles, medical director at the Catawba Care Christopher Clinic.

Courtesy of Dr. Craig Charles

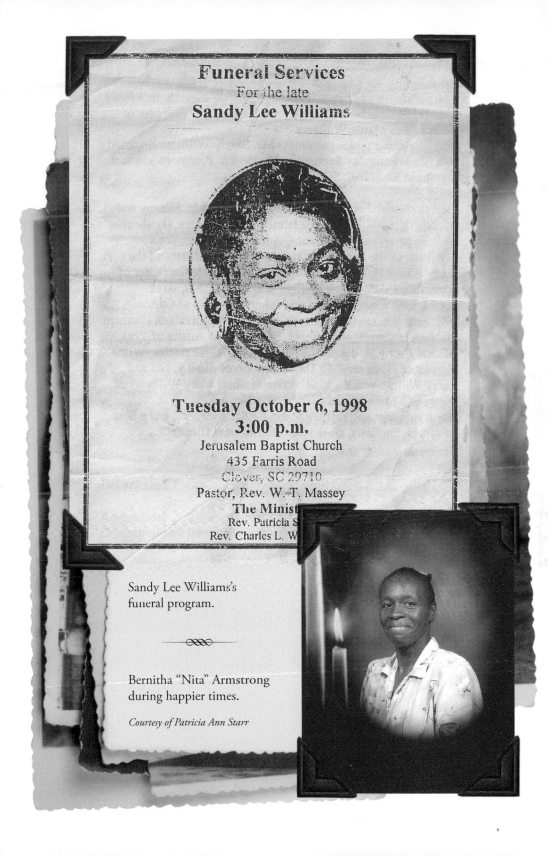

Funeral Services
For the late
Sandy Lee Williams

Tuesday October 6, 1998
3:00 p.m.
Jerusalem Baptist Church
435 Farris Road
Clover, SC 29710
Pastor, Rev. W. T. Massey
The Minist
Rev. Patricia S
Rev. Charles L. W

Sandy Lee Williams's
funeral program.

⟫⟫⟫

Bernitha "Nita" Armstrong
during happier times.

Courtesy of Patricia Ann Starr

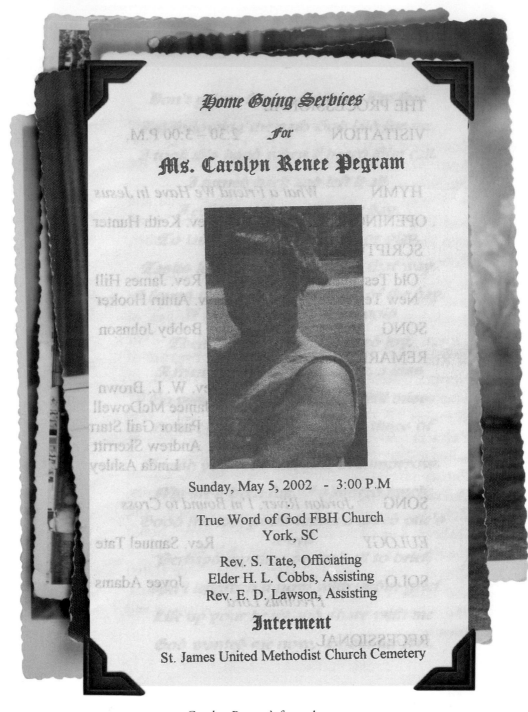

Home Going Services

for

Ms. Carolyn Renee Pegram

Sunday, May 5, 2002 - 3:00 P.M

True Word of God FBH Church
York, SC

Rev. S. Tate, Officiating
Elder H. L. Cobbs, Assisting
Rev. E. D. Lawson, Assisting

Interment

St. James United Methodist Church Cemetery

Carolyn Pegram's funeral program.
Generations Funeral Home buried many of Clover's residents who died of AIDS.

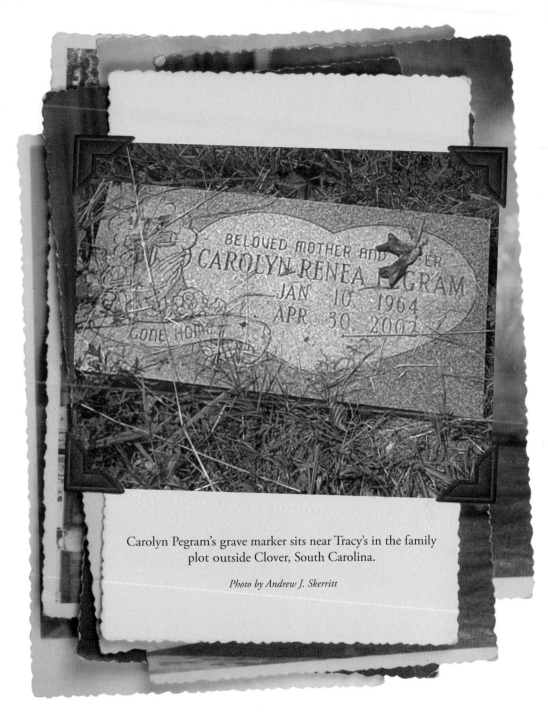

BELOVED MOTHER AND ...ER
CAROLYN RENEA PEGRAM
JAN 10 1964
APR 30 2002
GONE HOME

Carolyn Pegram's grave marker sits near Tracy's in the family plot outside Clover, South Carolina.

Photo by Andrew J. Skerritt

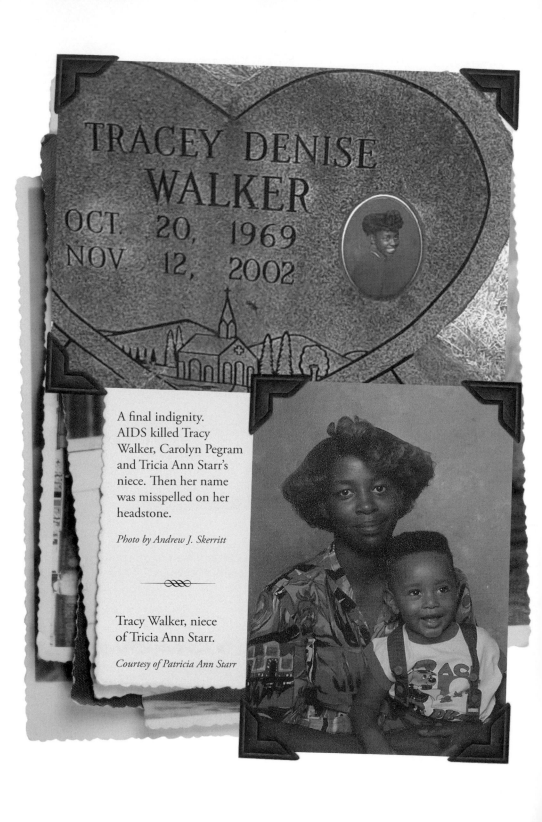

TRACEY DENISE
WALKER
OCT. 20, 1969
NOV. 12, 2002

A final indignity.
AIDS killed Tracy
Walker, Carolyn Pegram
and Tricia Ann Starr's
niece. Then her name
was misspelled on her
headstone.

Photo by Andrew J. Skerritt

❦

Tracy Walker, niece
of Tricia Ann Starr.

Courtesy of Patricia Ann Starr

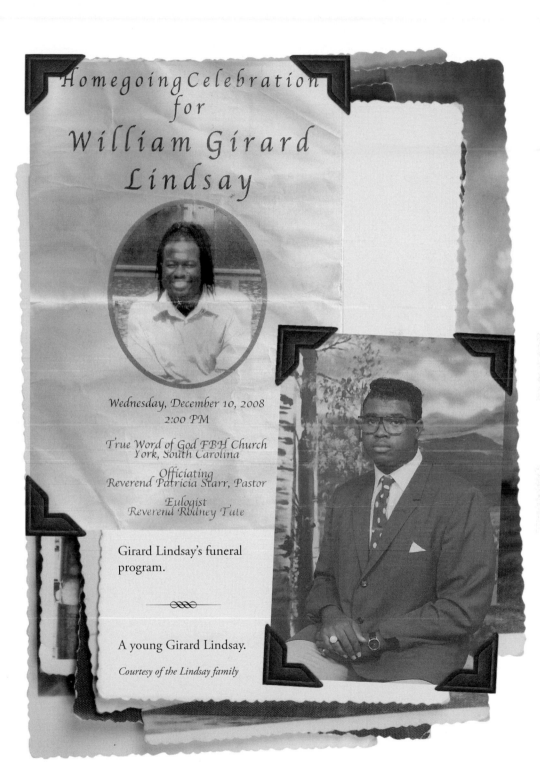

Homegoing Celebration
for
William Girard Lindsay

Wednesday, December 10, 2008
2:00 PM

True Word of God FBH Church
York, South Carolina

Officiating
Reverend Patricia Starr, Pastor

Eulogist
Reverend Rodney Tate

Girard Lindsay's funeral program.

A young Girard Lindsay.

Courtesy of the Lindsay family

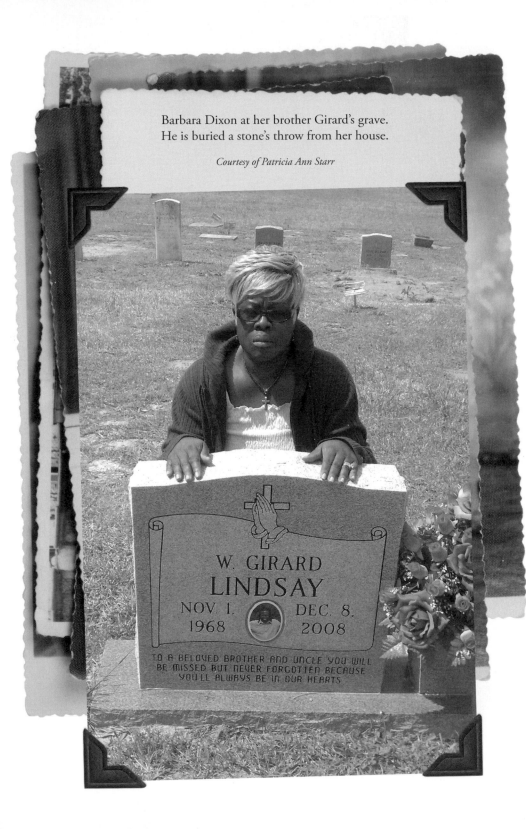

Barbara Dixon at her brother Girard's grave.
He is buried a stone's throw from her house.

Courtesy of Patricia Ann Starr

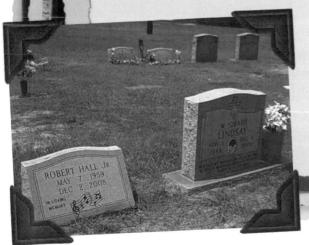

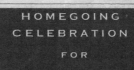

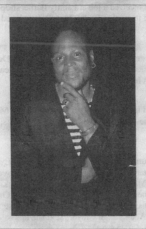

HOMEGOING CELEBRATION

FOR

MR. ROBERT HALL JR.

TRUEWORD OF GOD F.B.H. CHURCH
YORK, SOUTH CAROLINA

SATURDAY— DECEMBER 6, 2008
2:00 P.M.
REVEREND PATRICIA STARR-OFFICIATING

Robbie Hall's funeral program.

Robert Hall Jr. and Girard Lindsay were both claimed by AIDS a week apart. In death, they rest eternally side by side in Clover's black cemetery.

Photo by Andrew J. Skerritt

hidden eyes turned in her direction, necks craned through kitchen windows, and heads poked against screen doors as curious neighbors strained to catch a glimpse of this stranger in their midst. The only kind of white people who ventured down Queensgate Road were authority figures—sheriff's deputies, Clover police officers, social workers, teachers looking for the parents of delinquent students—or folks on the bottom—crack whores or redneck junkies craving a fix. People must have wondered about this woman who walked up Tricia Ann's driveway and knocked on the front door. When Tricia Ann answered the door, she found herself face-to-face with a white woman with short hair, glasses that were lodged between high cheekbones, and friendly, languid eyes that smiled easily.

As Tricia Ann sized up her guest, she didn't just see a white woman whose presence symbolized the curse afflicting the Pegram family. Tricia Ann could not have known or even imagined then that tragedy had conspired to bring Linda Ashley to her doorstep. And she would never have guessed that after their first uneasy encounter the relationship between them, client and social worker, would blossom into an unshakeable friendship: one woman conservatively religious, the other liberal; one black, the other white; both southern and both blessed with boundless reserves of empathy and compassion that would be vital as they each sought to understand the nature of the plague called AIDS.

While Tricia Ann lived within a stone's throw of where she grew up, Linda Ashley was at least five hours away from her hometown. Her mother's family roots were buried three generations deep in the soil of Duval County in what is now greater Jacksonville. Her maternal grandparents owned a decent-sized farmstead. Her grandfather, Percy Harold, raised cattle and grew vegetables to make the family self-sufficient. He cut logs and deployed a logging team to supply posts for the first electric lines in Duval County and all along the northeastern end of Florida.

Percy was a man of the outdoors. His wife was accustomed to him being gone two or three weeks at a time. Whenever Percy came home, though, he made his time there count. His wife bore him nine children. Harriette, Linda's mother, was the fifth, the middle child.

Linda's paternal grandfather worked for Erie Oil Company. His wife was Minorcan, a descendant of the Mediterranean indentured servants who were shipped to colonial Florida in 1768 as part of a plan by Dr. Andrew Turnbull to populate an area just south of St. Augustine. A strong, olive-skinned woman, Grandma Ashley was raised poor but was taught to think that she was as good as anyone else. Linda Ashley's father, Walter Clifford "Jack" Ashley, was dark complexioned and had black eyes. He named himself Jack when he was five years old, and they called him that from then on. Soon after he was drafted into the army, he married Harriette Harold. There was just enough time for the ceremony and a quick honeymoon before he sailed to Europe to fight Hitler and Mussolini.

When he returned from the war years later, like thousands of GIs of his generation, Sergeant Jack Ashley was reticent to talk about the horror and the bloodshed he witnessed. He'd say, "War is not pretty." Jack Ashley confined his memories and his medals to a wooden box on his closet shelf.

The three years that Jack Ashley was away fighting in Europe must have seemed like an eternity to his wife as she waited to start a family. Her husband had started to build a house before he left, but while he was on active duty, his wife was a nomad. Harriette stayed with one sister, then another. Sometimes she visited to help with a newborn baby or when she was just lonely and missed Jack. Armistice Day dawned on May 8, 1945. The war in Europe was over; Hitler had been vanquished. Before the end of that month, Jack was honorably discharged so he could return to his anxious bride.

Linda arrived April 25, 1947, on the crest of the baby boom that transformed postwar America. Linda entered a world trying to regain its equilibrium after the horrors of the previous eight years. Americans tried to laugh again and to forget the past. Even as Harriette Ashley nursed her day-old baby, her friends and neighbors in Jacksonville were traipsing off to movie theaters to watch Walt Disney's *Tom and Jerry*. But beneath the levity, southern towns like Jacksonville began to feel the rising tension of inevitable social change. Black GIs returning from Europe were unwilling to return to their subservient status. They had fought and won freedom overseas; they wanted to enjoy it at home. And white America had begun to respond to the swelling aspirations of its black citizens. Weeks before Linda's birth, Jackie Robinson, a talent from south Georgia, signed a contract with the Brooklyn Dodgers, making him the first African American in major-league baseball. That small opening signaled a sea change in American cultural and political life. It was a heady time.

As their firstborn, Linda enjoyed her parents' undivided attention for three years before a baby brother arrived, and when she was nine, a second brother was born into the Ashley household. Another two years elapsed before Harriette returned to the hospital delivery room to give birth to a baby girl. By then, Linda was eleven.

Linda remembers her childhood as an endless, idyllic summer. Her father loved the outdoors. The family spent many weekends camping out. He loved the water and taught his kids to swim early. With all the water around them—St. Johns River, Lake George, and the Atlantic Ocean—that was just being smart. But one of the first lessons Floridian children learn is that where there is fresh water, gators are usually close by. Once in a while, Linda saw them, but she never worried about the man-eating reptiles. She and her siblings were much more scared of another crawling reptile: snakes. Water moccasins and rattlers were a constant threat. But that didn't discourage the Ashley quartet from their outdoor adventures. They hardly ever wore shoes but preferred to ramble barefoot in the woods. They spent endless hours with both sets of grandparents. They especially loved to visit Ella and Percy at the farm. Linda liked to watch the cattle and play with her cousins. Each fall her grandparents butchered hogs and cooked sugarcane juice until it turned into thick, brown syrup. Linda never forgot the aroma of juice boiling all day over an open fire.

Childhood was wonderful. Then Linda became a teenager. In the summer of 1962, as she anticipated her freshman year at Dupont High School, Linda and her mother drove around in the family station wagon singing along to Bobby Vinton's "Roses Are Red" and Brenda Lee's "Break It to Me

Gently." As she blossomed into young adulthood, Linda's head filled with big dreams. She didn't want to be a stay-at-home mother; she wanted to attend college and become a teacher.

Linda's excitement during her first weeks of high school was soon over-shadowed by concerns that stretched far beyond the south side of Jacksonville. Saber rattling between the Soviet Union's Nikita Khrushchev and President John F. Kennedy turned into a nuclear standoff. The Cuban Missile Crisis gave Linda's mother's life new purpose. As tensions mounted in October 1962, she served as a designated driver for emergency evacuation drills. Teachers assigned each student a dog tag, lined them up in single file, loaded them into the car, and drove in a circle around the school. In the event of a nuclear attack, Harriette was supposed to load the children into her white station wagon and drive them to the potato barns for shelter.

"Now we know we would all have died before we got there," Linda says in hindsight. "Then we didn't know that. We were scared to death of Cuba." They took the drills seriously. If the Russians attacked, Jacksonville would've been a target. Five naval bases sat within a fifty-mile radius of the city.

The Cuban Missile Crisis interrupted the sweet pop music of Linda's high school life like a scratched record. But normal life soon returned and so did the fun. On weekends, she and her friends rode to the Jacksonville Beach or farther south to Daytona Beach, where they frolicked for endless hours on the sand and surf unfettered by adult concerns. Earlier on, Linda was just a shy, self-conscious girl among a group of hormone-crazed teenagers. Freshman and sophomore years came and went, and Linda had never ventured on a real date. But during junior year, a cousin conspired to change that.

It started with a blind date. Friends were headed to Jacksonville Beach and asked Linda to ride along. The group drove in her cousin Charlotte's car singing along to "Blue Velvet" and "Surfin' U.S.A."

Her date, Hugh, stood strong, handsome, and self-assured. As soon as they returned from the beach outing, he pursued her; he called her every day on the phone. That summer Linda blossomed into sweet sixteen, and her cheeks burned with the excitement that comes with attention from an older man.

But no father welcomed this kind of attention. Linda's father, Jack Ashley, would have disapproved if he had known about his daughter's suitor. Hugh looked old enough to have already graduated from high school, even college. Someone told her that her new boyfriend was about twenty-one, five years older than Linda. He was actually ten years older. And that wasn't all—he had a marital history. Hugh had an ex-wife and two children.

At first, Linda's parents were reluctant for their oldest child to start dating, so most of Linda and Hugh's early dates were disguised as group outings. Eventually they relented and allowed Linda to go out with Hugh unchaperoned. In retrospect, that fateful decision, one she celebrated at the time, signaled the beginning of her downfall. Linda was a typical straight-A student: smart with books but naive about things of the world. Although she was in the eleventh grade, she had only two classes to complete, a history class and an English course, in order to graduate and head off to college. But her aspirations dissolved in passion as she and Hugh groped and smooched in the backseat of his '57 Chevy convertible.

After Linda and Hugh began having sex, she gained a strange self-confidence. Her body spoke the language of love as she went about her school day. She couldn't wait for the bell to ring to liberate her to spend all her free time with Hugh. Their sex was furtive, passionate, and unprotected. It never occurred to Linda that she'd end up pregnant like her boyfriend's ex-wife. Times were different. The birth control pill had been introduced several years earlier, but it was prescribed for married women, not high school teenagers. Somehow, Linda never had the birds and bees conversation with anyone. In the early 1960s, sex education consisted of a black and white newsreel shown at school. During the lesson, teachers segregated the boys from the girls; each group watched the film giggling in separate rooms.

It wasn't surprising then that sixteen-year-old Linda never made the connection between the fun she and Hugh enjoyed in the backseat of his car and those grainy movies. Later, as a social worker, she noticed a similar ignorance among those young people who had been exposed to AIDS. "It never occurs to them," she says. "It never comes into their thought process."

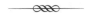

About two months after Linda and Hugh began fooling around, she awoke one morning feeling sick. The naive schoolgirl thought she had caught the flu. By the fourth day of getting out of bed and rushing to the toilet, she still hadn't figured it out. "I was in the bathroom throwing up my toenails," she recalled. Her mother noticed her discomfort. After all, Harriette Ashley had been pregnant at least four times in her life. So she asked Linda directly: "Is there any chance that you might be pregnant?"

That was never going to be a simple question. Those words coming from her mother's mouth must have hit Linda like a wind gust from an Atlantic hurricane on Jacksonville Beach. She couldn't muster a yes or a no. Her mother's wisdom knifed through her teenage naïveté and forced Linda to confront the cruel truth. She broke down crying. "It hadn't dawned on me at all," she said years later. "I had no idea."

The realization hit mother and daughter immediately: once Linda's pregnancy became public knowledge, the authorities would kick her out of school. She would subject her family to no end of gossip and shame. Her college dreams sailed right out the window. It was the longest term of her life, but Linda somehow managed to make it through the rest of eleventh grade keeping her pregnancy a secret. She carried her books in front of her stomach; she wore baggy clothes that hid her protruding bump. Linda felt powerless, as if life had conspired to rob her of all her once-happy choices.

But her parents, Jack and Harriette, knew exactly what to do. They ordered Hugh over to the house. When he arrived, the four—mother, father, pregnant daughter, and boyfriend—sat in the backyard on lawn chairs. Jack Ashley didn't bother with small talk. He went straight to the point. "She's pregnant," he said. "What are you going to do about it?" Jack Ashley's intentions were clear. He didn't want his daughter disgraced by having a child out of wedlock.

Linda and Hugh made up their minds that night. They decided to elope. One weekend that spring, they drove north to Folkston, Georgia, exchanged vows in front of a justice of the peace, and then returned that Saturday night for the Dupont High junior prom.

By then, Linda's protruding midsection couldn't be disguised. She was visibly pregnant. That fall she enrolled in adult education classes to earn her GED. But the first day she walked into her new school, the atmosphere depressed her. Linda felt as if she had been unjustly sentenced to a room full of dumb kids. Her thoughtless sexual fling had brought her as low as those former schoolmates she once looked down upon. To escape, she convinced the teacher to let her read the textbook at home and take the exams to get a real diploma. And so the straight-A student who once dreamed of graduating at the top of the Dupont High Class of 1965 with a diploma instead walked across the stage at the Duval County School District central office to collect her Central Adult Education Diploma.

While everyone else shopped and frantically decorated their homes on Christmas Eve 1964, a sixteen-year-old lay on a bed in Baptist Medical Center, her once lithe body wracked by waves of pain that emanated from somewhere near her belly button and slowly pinged every nerve from the soles of her feet to the top of her head. To her former classmates consumed by revelry, Linda was an afterthought. She felt alone. She was alone. "I was scared to death."

Back then, doctors and nurses prevented anyone but the mother from being in the delivery room. So Linda lay on her back listening to the tick-tock of the clock on the wall like a hammer pulsing inside her brain. She tried to time her contractions as each wave of pain rippled through her midsection. But the effect was agony, not serenity. To distract herself, she asked the attending nurse for a magazine to read.

Giving birth in the mid-'60s, with women being put to sleep with general anesthesia, seems rather crude compared with modern methods. There was no father in the delivery room capturing it all with a video camera. Linda doesn't remember much about giving birth except for the frantic efforts of doctors and nurses as they tried to stanch her internal hemorrhaging. That night she lost five pints of blood. She almost died.

Joey arrived kicking and wailing on Christmas Eve 1964. His relieved mother thought he looked gorgeous with his olive skin and a snowy cap of beautiful hair. Although he had been shielded from the tropical Florida sun for nine months, the newborn looked as if he had been conceived and incubated on sunny Jacksonville Beach.

But if Linda's son Joey was a delight, his father was a disaster. Hugh came blessed with arms and shoulders like a football player and a healthy disrespect for his young wife. He had grown up poor near Brunswick, Georgia, but quickly learned that a man with skillful hands could easily carve a path out of poverty. At the time he married Linda, Hugh worked as a machine operator in a boxboard plant. But he didn't just bring home a paycheck. Each day he stepped over the threshold he subjected his stay-at-home teen bride to a bucketful of abuse. In those pre-confessional, pre–*Dr. Phil* days, a wife didn't tell anyone if her husband was abusive. Shame bought her silence; fear sealed her lips.

Hugh was the sole breadwinner of the family, and he never let his wife forget that he was the boss. He gained even more control after he uprooted his family from their familiar Jacksonville surroundings and headed to Hendersonville in the western North Carolina mountains. Around that time, his drinking escalated, and he began to struggle at work. He wasn't cut out to be a supervisor, and he was miserable. His unhappiness on the job spilled over at home. Eventually he quit, and the family returned to Jacksonville. Joey was about three at the time, and Linda felt he was old enough for day care. Linda went to work for the first time, as a secretary at Gulf Life Insurance. She felt liberated from a life of subservience and underappreciated domesticity. Later she carried her newfound confidence and growing clerical skills to a chiropractic group. But Linda didn't linger in the clerical pool for too long. One day, after she heard about a vacancy at WJXT, the local Post-Newsweek television station, she saw a chance to use the smarts she had tucked away since her senior year in high school. She called the personnel director every two weeks to check for job openings until she relented.

"She hired me to get me off her back," Linda says. In those days, even without a college degree, a young white woman could climb the corporate ladder if she worked hard enough. She started as the lowest clerk in the office and rose to the station's assistant business manager in ten years. But as her career blossomed, Linda's marriage disintegrated in a never-ending replay of drunken, ill-tempered insults and put-downs. "I thought if I could cook better or if I could get prettier it would get better, but it never did," she said later.

In public, Hugh played the nice guy, but the minute he came home he turned as mean as a rattlesnake. Each time she felt like leaving and going back home to her parents, she would hear her grandmother's words ring in her head: "You made your bed, and you have to lie in it." Old-fashioned puritan guilt boxed her in. This was fitting punishment for her teenage foolishness. Her husband grew increasingly abusive. He cussed and fussed, his rages fueled by Crown Royal and domestic beer. "Then he'd try to make love to me," she said.

One weekend he got pretty drunk, slurring his words, staggering around the house. The odor of stale liquor assailed her nostrils. It turned her stomach and made her want to vomit. She'd had enough. She was leaving.

The sound of that threat sobered up Hugh in a hurry. He became sputtering mad. He rushed into the bedroom and pulled a shotgun out of the closet. "Nobody is gonna git my wife and my son," he yelled. He threatened to kill Linda, Joey, and then himself. He didn't follow through, but Linda couldn't have known that her husband's threat would hang over their son.

Linda refused to wait for Hugh to summon enough drunken courage to carry out his threat. She grabbed her son, ran out of the house, and never looked back.

Hugh's response to his wife's hasty departure surprised even her: he ended up in the hospital. Linda learned about his condition soon afterward when a doctor called her on Hugh's behalf. "You need to stay with him," he urged. "He needs you."

But she was adamant. "I'm not going back," she told him. "I'm not putting my son at risk. I'm not putting myself at risk." Within months she had bought a house on the south side of Jacksonville. She didn't ask for alimony. Hugh was supposed to pay forty dollars a week in child support, but he never did until the court stepped in and garnished his wages. Once he started paying child support, however, Hugh demanded his parental rights. He wanted to see Joey every other weekend, even though he didn't know what to do with the boy during those father and son get-togethers.

Hugh's fatherly instinct ebbed and flowed depending on his social life. "When he got his first girlfriend, he started leaving us alone," Linda said. "The only time we heard from him was when he got a new girlfriend and wanted to show Joey off." As her son grew older, Joey learned the rules of having divorced parents. If he could fulfill his father's social needs, then his father could take care of Joey's material needs. The father-son bond, often so strong and selfless, morphed into a users' relationship. When Joey wanted money, he called his father. If Hugh wanted to show off Joey to one of his girlfriends, he came to get him. Sometimes on the weekends, father and son headed for the beach. While Hugh drank at the bar on the boardwalk with friends, Joey rambled on the beach all afternoon; at nightfall he crawled into his father's car to sleep.

After she turned thirty, Linda was content. She was independent. Life was stable. Her job at the television station paid good money. She loved working for the Post-Newsweek station, which used a computer system made by Jefferson-Pilot Communications. Around that time, however, she heard about a vacant software customer service position at the North Carolina–based company. At first she was hesitant to apply, but a girlfriend convinced her she could learn the software system pretty quickly. It was 1984. Joey was grown and lived on his own. Linda felt unconstrained. She relocated to the Carolinas.

Working for Jefferson-Pilot gave Linda a freedom she had never imagined. Her job took her all over the country. During those years, she fulfilled her lifelong dream of seeing some of the places she had read about in high school. If she flew out West, for example, she'd stay over for the weekend so she could visit the Arizona desert and national parks.

Meanwhile, as Linda thrived, her son struggled to find his way. He couldn't seem to hold a job for long. He was moody and brooding. After a long phone conversation, he agreed to come to live with his mother in Rock Hill, South Carolina. The new arrangement took getting used to. Linda had come to relish the freedom of having her own space. She treasured her solitude. But she was willing to sacrifice her comfort for the sake of her only child. As soon as he found a job, he'd move out and live on his own.

That was the way Joey was. He was Linda's wild child. Soon he found a girlfriend. He spent more time at her place than at his. At last, Joey, the troubled son from an equally troubled union, seemed to have found happiness. So Linda thought.

While Linda was away on business in Winston-Salem, North Carolina, she heard a knock on her hotel room door. As she opened the door, she expected to see hotel staff offering towels. But it wasn't. It was two of her closest friends. The look on their faces foretold their horrific news. "Joey. Oh my god," Linda screamed.

Distraught over a breakup with his girlfriend, her son had shot himself.

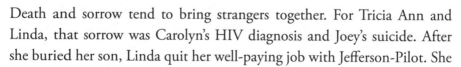

Death and sorrow tend to bring strangers together. For Tricia Ann and Linda, that sorrow was Carolyn's HIV diagnosis and Joey's suicide. After she buried her son, Linda quit her well-paying job with Jefferson-Pilot. She felt compelled to start over.

Two decades earlier, her pregnancy with Joey had killed her college dreams, but now his death gave them rebirth. She enrolled in York County Technical College. She no longer wanted to teach; she would become a social worker who helped those who hurt.

15

AIDS LADY

Linda's college education was more a sprint than a casual walk as she tried to make up for decades of lost time—twelve months at York Technical College, then a bachelor's degree at Winthrop University in 1995. She spent the next year commuting from Rock Hill to the University of South Carolina in Columbia, pursuing a master's degree in social work.

When she was a college student, Linda believed her calling was hospice care—providing comfort to those who were grieving and dying just like she had once grieved. Instead, after graduating in May 1996, Linda found herself walking into the red brick York County Health Department for an interview to be the HIV/AIDS case manager.

Fifteen years after the first reported case of acquired immune deficiency syndrome, York County still lacked any cohesive response to the epidemic. At that time, 289 people in the county had been diagnosed with HIV, and many of them were already dead. Cliff Caldwell was cremated just weeks before Linda took the job. Young men and women were dying in shame and there was nothing but a halfhearted official response. The case manager in charge of AIDS worked part-time before she left on maternity leave. After the baby she wasn't coming back. A grant from the Regional AIDS Consortium, a group of a dozen counties around Charlotte-Mecklenburg, paid her salary. Linda's assignment meant that she had to go up to Charlotte to the Regional Consortium meeting with case managers from ten other neighboring counties. It offered her the opportunity to talk to people who were doing similar jobs. She also had to drive ninety miles south to the state Department of Health and Environmental Control in Columbia for more meetings.

In the mid-1990s, while medical professionals nationwide embraced the introduction of protease inhibitors in the battle against HIV and AIDS, the York County Health Department played catch-up. Local physicians were largely unprepared to treat people with AIDS. Some called Dr. Ball in Columbia for advice on prescriptions and treatment regimens. York County, with a population of over one hundred thousand people, did not have a full-time infectious disease specialist. The county health department lacked the money to adequately care for people with AIDS, most of whom were poor and uninsured. No one applied for the six-figure grants made available through the Ryan White CARE Act. Those rendered disabled from HIV and AIDS struggled to find decent housing and to pay for prescription drugs that cost around $10,000 a year.

Early on, Linda recognized that Dr. Ball, then the state epidemiologist, was an invaluable asset for small-town caseworkers like her. If you had local doctors who didn't know what they were doing or knew nothing about the meds, you could ask Ball to call them for a consult. He'd instruct the doctors for free.

"The local doctors had no idea; they didn't know how to diagnose it," Linda says. "They didn't know what medications to prescribe. Some of them were as scared of the patients as anyone else." Dr. Ball was the person, along with STD/AIDS director Lynda Kettinger, who flew to Washington to fight for AIDS funding for his state. He could speak authoritatively about AIDS when few others in the state could.

At a seminar Linda attended, Ball lectured about protease inhibitors. He was a slight man. He wore glasses and looked like a rich white guy just off the golf course. He spoke with that wonderful Charleston accent that said he obviously came from money. People listened to him. He was smooth.

While protease inhibitors were introduced in 1995 and were being prescribed in the big cities, it took another several years for local physicians in Rock Hill to start prescribing the more potent, effective drugs. "In the beginning, all we had was AZT," Linda says. "When the new stuff came out, nobody knew what to do."

Ball did. He knew what to prescribe, what was acceptable, and what was in clinical trials. Back then, there were usually no drug trials in rural areas. "You had to be in the big city," Linda says.

Even as a case manager, Linda soon learned the calculus of AIDS: CD4 counts told how the immune system was holding up and how much of the virus was in the blood. Every person has a CD4 count that tells whether the immune system is healthy or not. A CD4 count from eight hundred to twelve hundred is in the healthy range. Then scientists introduced the viral load test, which would tell how many particles of the human immunodeficiency virus there were to a unit of blood. It would tell how sick a patient was and how the virus was progressing in his body. If the person with AIDS could get the viral load under control, then he could extend his life. But money was a stumbling block. At the time, a viral load test cost $350, and it had to be done every ninety days. "A lot of rural doctors had no idea what the test was, and they didn't know how to read it," Linda says.

The health department couldn't force a person to be tested even if a contact gave them names of people exposed to AIDS. Another social worker, the designated STD tracker, drove around to contact people named as sexual partners by those being treated for syphilis, gonorrhea, and chlamydia. Linda dealt strictly with people who had tested HIV positive or had full-blown AIDS symptoms. The health department provided supervision and an office to keep the thirty-two names of known HIV/AIDS cases under lock and key.

The minute she was hired, she dove headlong into the job. Within six months her caseload more than doubled. In December 1996, she had seventy-three names in her files. DHEC records show that forty-one people were diagnosed with HIV in her three-county district that year. Of those, twenty-nine lived in York County. And tiny Clover had more than its fair share.

When Linda walked into the county health department as a naive social worker in May 1996, she encountered Faye Ballard, the HIV nurse. Ballard was an experienced nurse. She not only provided care for people who showed up at the health department, she was also on hand for the York County AIDS Task Force annual weekend retreats for people with AIDS. Linda felt kind of intimidated. It didn't help that initially Ballard wasn't very welcoming. "I don't know why they hired a social worker," she told Linda one day. "I have been doing this stuff anyway." But after a few months, as she observed Linda's hustle, Ballard's attitude changed.

"She saw the craziness. She finally came in one day and said, 'I guess social workers are OK.'"

Ballard's job was to give HIV diagnoses. And she had been doing it for a while. People came in for tests and waited a week for the results before they returned to see her. "When you had a positive, she hated it," Linda says.

One day a young woman in her early twenties came in for her test results. She was HIV positive. "The girl went to pieces," Linda says. "She threatened to kill herself." In a panic, Ballard knocked on Linda's office door. She was afraid the distraught girl might actually take her own life.

"Linda, I need you now!"

"I went in there, and we worked together. When she left, we had a plan."

Their professional bond was cemented that day. "When Faye did that, I knew I had made the grade," Linda says. Three years later, when Linda left the county health department to open an AIDS clinic, Ballard was one of the first people she tried to hire. Later Ballard joined the staff and became the best nurse the Christopher Clinic ever had.

To be an effective case manager, Linda had to gain the trust of the people she was paid to help. She had to learn to be tactful. When she talked to people with HIV, they would usually be embarrassed and reluctant to openly discuss drug reactions and symptoms. They might be dying of AIDS, but they didn't want anyone else to know. "They were afraid you were going to tell somebody else," she says.

Visits to Tricia Ann's Cloverdale neighborhood offered the kind of challenge only a person schooled in espionage would appreciate. Several people with AIDS lived close enough to see who came and went to one another's homes. Sometimes Linda had to borrow someone else's car so as not to give herself away. Whenever Linda's health department vehicle pulled up in front of a certain house, Tricia Ann's phone would begin to ring.

"A white lady is going into Jim's house. What happened, is he sick? Does he got it?" the inquisitive caller would ask. That white woman was usually Linda.

"You can tell social workers," Tricia Ann says. The first thing Linda did was get out and put her purse in the trunk of her car, in full view of all the hidden eyes that watched her arrival. As Tricia Ann looked outside at the woman, she shook her head. "That's the worse thing you can do. You are saying 'Rob me.' It's saying you have money. I told her to stop doing that."

Linda walked up to the front door holding a folder with some paperwork. Tricia Ann answered the door and invited her inside but was initially skeptical of the visitor. Experience had taught her very little good came of black-white interactions.

Linda had grown up among mostly white folks in rural Jacksonville. But she was open-minded. She wanted to feel at home. "She was trying to be one of us," Tricia Ann says, but her body language was wrong. When Tricia Ann's sons entered the house, Linda would exchange slang with them.

"We would just look at her and burst out laughing," Tricia Ann says. "She just tried to be hip." She told Linda, "You can't be black, so stop trying." That candid talk across the color line and their mutual concern for Carolyn forged a bond between the two women. "We got close," Tricia Ann says. "She was OK. I could talk to her. She was going to have problems, more than she could imagine, dealing with this neighborhood."

This wasn't just a minor inconvenience. The only white women who came into the neighborhood were usually social workers. If nobody in the house was sick and nobody was on welfare, then who was that white woman, and why was she in that house? Tricia Ann had to field these kinds of questions from her neighbors.

If people didn't learn to trust Linda, then they wouldn't trust the health department to test and treat them for HIV and AIDS. As the two women got to know each other better, Tricia Ann tried to educate Linda about the obstacles she faced. The biggest hurdles were her race and that she was an outsider. Tricia Ann was black and lived in the neighborhood. If Linda tried too hard, the walls of resistance would be erected higher. She couldn't just try to fit in. People had to let her in. "They have to learn to trust you," Tricia Ann told her. For southern black folks that has never been easy.

"You're dealing with a disease that people are going to talk about," Tricia Ann says. Once Linda was identified as the "AIDS lady," everyone she spoke to in public, every house she visited, would be tainted. Serving people who desperately needed medical care in Cloverdale required a very different approach from the one she used in a larger town like Rock Hill. Linda, for her part, was concerned that once Tricia Ann became involved with AIDS outreach, she would face similar obstacles. "They are going to think that way about you," she told the black woman. But Tricia Ann brushed that talk aside.

"No," she said. "I live in this neighborhood. I am a pastor. I'm always going in and out. I didn't just wait until now." Linda needed to know how to reach the people. She had the names of those infected and where they lived, but that didn't get her foot inside the door. "I said, 'Linda, they're not going to let you into their house.'"

Timing was half the problem. "Linda had to learn that when Cliff died and left the list, that rocked Clover," Tricia Ann says. News of the list spread quickly. Rumors flew. Anyone with a bad cough or a skin rash came under suspicion.

Linda's first task was to establish street cred. Once Tricia Ann allowed Linda into her house, others walls in Cloverdale might begin to crumble. "She had to trust somebody. I was in the neighborhood," Tricia Ann says. Many of Tricia Ann's neighbors didn't have private health insurance, so most of them went to the health department for all their maladies—flu, sore throats, even STDs. AIDS presented a much higher hurdle. "They were definitely not going to visit the health department and take the chance of being seen," Tricia Ann said years later. "And no way Linda was going to bring a nurse to their home."

Together the two women found a way. They tested people in the woods near Rose Hill Cemetery, Clover's white burial ground, and at churches. They met people wherever they were; they took every offer, ventured into every venue, to talk about how AIDS was killing young people in Clover.

Social workers who deal with welfare mothers expect to attend a court hearing occasionally. But social workers who counsel people with AIDS attend funerals. And for Linda, attending African American funerals was a surprising cultural excursion. "I went to more funerals in that first year in that job than I did in my whole life," she said later.

White and black southern folks bury their dead differently, she soon learned. She remembers her first African American AIDS funeral. She was totally unaware that such events were like an open-mike afternoon mixed in with a camp meeting. They went on for hours. Linda didn't anticipate all the weeping, clapping, and singing. She was struck by the sight of the women who wore white nurse-like uniforms and white gloves and ran around fanning people who fell out in the aisles.

One of her first African American funerals was for a young woman who had died of AIDS. When Linda had met her, the young woman drank too much liquor and took too few of her meds. Her sister was a minister, and she was the black sheep of the family. She was a tiny little thing when she died. With so many deaths over the years, it was hard for Linda to remember the details of each one. But some images are unforgettable. The dead woman had two children; one was a little boy about ten years old. At the funeral he wore a suit that was at least two sizes too big. The casket sat open during the service. At the end, someone came over, took the boy by the hand, and led him to the casket. He was assigned to cover his mother and close the top of the casket.

"I thought it was the most cruel and heartless thing to do to a child," Linda says. "But for them, it was a tradition."

16

SANDY

The cars began to arrive early that Tuesday afternoon, October 6, 1998. The sun still bore its early autumn sting. Leaves were still green. But, as the old folks say, the green leaves fall as well as the yellow ones. And mourners converged on Jerusalem Baptist Church on Farris Road to bury Sandy Lee Williams, one of the green leaves that had fallen from the tree. She lived hard and fast and died young. She was only twenty-nine, but she left behind four young motherless children, two boys and two girls.

Jerusalem Baptist is an old, redbrick, Victorian-type structure with two steeples on top, a black-painted bell out front, and a cemetery out back. It sits south of town amid the wide expanses of farmland where Clover begins to give way to Smyrna and the western reaches of York County.

The funeral was scheduled to begin at three, early enough to force Sandy's girlhood friends to take the afternoon off from work to say good-bye to the woman who had died a week earlier after a "prolonged illness," as her funeral program said.

On that afternoon, Sandy's pastor, Reverend William T. "Dub" Massey, had company on the dais. Next to him sat Reverend Patricia Starr and Reverend Charles White. While Massey lived miles away in Rock Hill, Starr and White were Sandy's neighbors. They knew her from their involvement with the food pantry and their outreach to people afflicted with the plague coursing through black Clover.

The mourners, including Linda Ashley, packed the cushioned pews that afternoon. As they waited for the service to start, folks tried to stay cool fanning themselves with the Generation Funeral Home fans. The casket sat open in the front. Sandy, young as ever, her face made up, lay dressed in a pink gown with a matching pink carnation. As the processional sounded and the last few mourners filed in and filled the pews around the sanctuary, Massey spoke the invocation, his voice filling the room.

Massey, a former high school quarterback, had made a name for himself as a member of the Friendship Nine, a group of junior college students who chose jail instead of bail after they were arrested for lunch counter demonstrations in Rock Hill during the early 1960s. As a soldier of the civil rights movement, he had fought for a better life for future generations of black folks. But, invoking God's name over Sandy's lifeless body, Massey must have felt pain and disappointment in his heart to see a once-hopeful future destroyed by the scourge of drugs and AIDS.

Sandy was born on April 18, 1969. She was the second youngest of six children. Unlike many of her neighbors, she grew up with her mother, Mattie, and father, Sammy, under the same roof. The year Sandy was born, college students were in full rebellion as they protested the war in Vietnam. Turmoil and unrest ruled the country. And Sandy seemed to have inherited that spirit of restlessness and rebellion. Early on, she chose her own path that led to the streets. She was also born with the curse of being beautiful too soon, friends and neighbors say. Her face leaps off the page of her funeral program; her full smile, even teeth, and plum-sized cheeks decorate her face like jewelry.

Grown men on the streets of Cloverdale began to lay traps for her long before she was old enough to understand the intricacies of love and lust. She was young, innocent, and very immature—easy prey for the two-legged wolves. She had long hair but wore it in a ponytail or a tight bun. She possessed the kind of elegant shape that made an ordinary pair of blue jeans look like velvet.

Her childhood friend Mia Howell remembers Sandy, her classmate from elementary school to middle school to junior high and high school.

Sandy was average; she didn't strive for As. Cs and Ds were good enough. She loved to laugh and enjoy herself. She was a free spirit. "Sandy was always walking in the rain with no shoes on," Mia says.

Sandy loved to have fun. Even as young as twelve or thirteen, Sandy and her friends got together to drink Schaeffer beer and Seagram's gin. They drank and laughed and danced and popped speed pills and acted crazy in an innocent teenage way. It seemed so natural. They desperately wanted to fit in, to be like everyone else.

While Sandy was still underage, her father often confronted the grown men he thought were too old to be with his daughter. He'd go out on the street and beg her to come home, the same way Tricia Ann and her brother John would beg Carolyn to get off the streets. But she ignored him. "She was going to live her life," Tricia Ann says. "No matter what anyone said, it wasn't going to change her. She wasn't going to stop."

Sandy never talked about her dreams with Mia. When the two got together, it was for the moment—thinking about the future was far too depressing. All they had to look forward to was working at a textile factory just like their parents. At thirteen years old, they tried to postpone the future by filling the present with hard liquor and speed. They weren't old enough to buy alcohol, but they were persuasive enough to find adults to buy it for them. If a wink and a smile weren't enough, they paid adults to buy their booze. Everybody else did it. It seemed like such a normal childhood in the 1980s. But the era of innocent fun had passed. Teenage indiscretions could turn deadly in the age of AIDS. As they grew older, they hung with the crowd at Black's Café and on the steps of Generation Funeral Home. But Sandy wasn't content with the gin and the beer and the pills. She soon graduated to more serious drugs and more adult company. Then her ponytail wasn't so neat any more; her jeans didn't quite fit the same way; her teeth became more eyesore than asset. She let herself go.

Sandy started to sleep with a lot of men in Clover. It wasn't for money. She knew it bothered her father, but she was defiant. She loved to have a good time, enjoyed the adulation of older men, and just didn't care about the consequences of her sexual behavior. "The old men in Cloverdale love them some Sandy, and Sandy loved her some old men," Tricia Ann often said. With her promiscuity, babies naturally followed. Sandy had her first girl when she was fifteen or sixteen and three more after that: four children, four baby daddies in all.

Sandy was about sixteen and still in high school when she was first diagnosed with HIV. She caught a cold she just couldn't shake. At first the nurse at the health department thought Sandy was pregnant. But tests soon showed a far worse condition. It may have shaken her for a moment, but it didn't drastically change the way Sandy lived. She possessed an untamed heart. Even as a teenage schoolgirl, Sandy used to slip out of her parents' home to spend time with the older men who never seemed to be able to resist that smile. It was a minor miracle that Sandy gave birth to four children without infecting any of them.

After she developed AIDS, her nice, well-shaped body shrunk to nothing. The teeth that once accessorized her pretty smile started decaying from drug use. To Linda, Carolyn was the toughest AIDS case. For Tricia Ann, Sandy was worse. "She fought us all along the way, then she would come back and say, 'I love you, Miss Tricia Ann.'" Sandy fought AIDS. And she fought those who cared for her, Tricia Ann says. She was determined to live her life on her terms no matter what.

Her final battle was with her parents and caregivers about taking her meds. One day in July 1998, Tricia Ann looked out her kitchen door and saw Sandy running and screaming, with her mother and father chasing right behind her. "Tell them I don't want to do it no more!' she screamed as she ran into Tricia Ann's house. Tricia Ann tried to remain calm amid the excitement.

"What's wrong, Sandy?"

"No. I don't want to take any more medicine!"

"She was telling them 'no.' It was sad. It was so funny the way she was just running, the way she refused to take the medicine."

When Mia started working after school, she and Sandy had lost touched with each other. They no longer sought fun in the same places. Mia moved to the other side of town while Sandy remained in the old neighborhood. But when Mia heard Sandy was sick and dying, she came looking for her former best friend in Piedmont Medical Center. Mia climbed into bed with Sandy, and they talked and they laughed about the crazy days in high school.

The day Sandy died, Wednesday, September 30, 1998, Tricia Ann was scheduled to clean houses for some white folks in Charlotte, a forty-minute drive from her home in Clover. That morning it took her considerably longer to reach the first house of the day because of rush hour traffic jams south of the city.

At 9:05 her cell phone rang. It was Sandy's mother. Sandy had been readmitted to the hospital. She refused to take her medicine. The family didn't want hospice. She had bedsores and had lost weight. She was deteriorating fast. They were giving her morphine, but she didn't want to take it; it made her sleep too much.

"They say something is wrong. I'm losing her. You have to come," Sandy's mother said.

"I can't. I have to clean today," Tricia Ann said. "Let me speak to the nurse." Tricia Ann asked the nurse what was wrong.

"She's dying. They just need to be prepared for that," she replied. As soon as she hung up, Tricia Ann muttered an excuse to her client, headed for her car, and drove straight to the hospital in Rock Hill. Sandy was on the hospice floor. Tricia Ann walked over to Sandy and held her hand.

"Do you know who I am?" she asked. Sandy, eyes barely open, shook her head. "Make sure you pray. You don't have to say it out loud. God knows the heart."

Every day Tricia Ann visited Sandy and went over the sinner's prayer, an evangelical plea for divine forgiveness, with her. The pastor in her refused to let Sandy go without settling all her outstanding business. She assured the dying woman that it was OK for her to leave. "You've made peace with your family. You can go home."

Sandy seemed to take her words to heart because she sighed deeply. Her eyes remained closed. Immediately, her mother became hysterical.

"Sandy, you can't leave me!"

At that point, a nurse walked in. "Where are the children?" she asked. "If they are going to see their mother alive they have to come now. She's dying."

Tricia Ann squeezed Sandy's hand, then let go and walked out of the room. While Sandy's mother went to collect the children to say their final good-byes, her father paced outside the hospital room, distraught. He was inconsolable. He took Sandy's death personally, as if he had failed her. But it wasn't his fault that his daughter was born beautiful and never quite learned to do more than share her good looks with men on the street. Sandy had made her own decisions.

As Tricia Ann walked out of Sandy's hospital room, she knew that it was the last time she would see Sandy alive. She knew Sandy would be dead by the time they returned; her children would arrive too late to say good-bye to their mother. And she was right. Almost two hours later, when they walked into Sandy's hospital room, someone whispered, "She's gone," as if afraid that the dead would hear and be insulted.

On hearing the news, Sandy's mother passed out.

"Sandy needed her mom to leave," Tricia Ann says. "She didn't need to be there. Her dad needed to be there." In tears, Sandy's father had retreated to a nearby conference room.

"I tried to get her to come home so many times," he sobbed.

"It broke my heart to see this grown man cry," Tricia Ann says. "But it wasn't his fault. Sandy made her choice."

With all of Sandy's numerous relatives, it took a week to arrange the funeral. The tragedy of Sandy's life and death is magnified when one considers that, even as she gave up hope and had surrendered her will to live, others who were equally sick with AIDS were doing quite the opposite.

The day Sandy was buried, the *New York Times* published an article, "Holding AIDS at Bay, Only to Face 'Lazarus Syndrome,'" about a forty-five-year-old New Yorker who was on death's door with lymphoma, mycobacterium avium complex, microsporidiosis, and esophageal thrush only to rebound thanks to the help of protease inhibitors, the anti-HIV compounds introduced two years earlier.

Why did Sandy die while the New Yorker lived? Was it because he had better medical care than she did? At the time of her death, protease inhibitors had begun to drastically reduce the mortality rate among people with HIV and AIDS in most of the country, the *New York Times* reported.

A Johns Hopkins University study showed that the new medicines had also reduced the number of AIDS-related opportunistic infections by more than 60 percent, according to the *New York Times* article. The numbers of people dying of AIDS had declined by 50 percent—in most of the country. But not where Sandy lived. The shame of having AIDS was still worse than the disease itself. And so, six days after she died, dozens of friends and relatives converged on Jerusalem Baptist to remember Sandy. That October afternoon, after Reverend Massey prayed the invocation, the Jerusalem Baptist choir filled the building with song. Folks rose in the pews, stomped their leather shoes, and sang and danced along with the music as if forgetting for a moment the reason for the gathering. Massey read the Old Testament lesson, and Reverend Charles White Jr. followed with the New Testament lesson.

As the last chords died, Reverend Starr stepped up to the pulpit. Baptist churches tend to be hostile to women speaking in their pulpits, but Dub Massey had no such reservations. Sandy had wanted Miss Tricia Ann to speak over her body. Miss Tricia Ann, as Sandy called her, had traveled the long, dark road of AIDS with Sandy from the beginning to the end.

Tricia Ann looked out into the crowded congregation of mourners. Sandy's two daughters and two sons were there, the youngest only five years old. Years later, when asked about his mother, he would barely remember the funeral. Near the front sat her mother, Mattie, and father, Sammy, who loved her more than anyone could imagine. There were her sisters and brothers. There was room enough for uncles and aunts and friends, a church full of people who loved Sandy but couldn't save her from herself. Looking out from the pulpit at Jerusalem Baptist Church, Tricia Ann eulogized Sandy, the daughter, sister, and mother. She wanted badly to say, "Sandy died of AIDS." She wanted to shout with all the air in her lungs that AIDS was killing the young people, but she couldn't. She had to honor the wishes of Sandy's grieving parents. Sandy died of sickle cell, not AIDS. After Sandy died, hers was the first name local AIDS activists wanted to put on the AIDS name quilt in Charlotte, North Carolina. But Sandy's family didn't want them to. After all, Sandy didn't die of AIDS; she had sickle cell.

And so instead, on that hot October afternoon, Tricia Ann preached about how we judge the outward appearance. "We are so quick to condemn and judge, but God knows the heart," she said. "There but for the grace of God go you or I. Don't be so quick to condemn this child. We all have children who have made mistakes. God is a good God. God is a forgiving God. We need to have compassion for people and examine our own selves and our families."

Tricia Ann remembers thinking there was a time when funerals were for burying old people but now "we are burying our young."

After Reverend Starr fell silent, Bobby Johnson sang another solo for Sandy before the six pallbearers walked alongside the casket as the staff from Generation Funeral Home wheeled the body outside to the burial ground. Before sundown, a fresh mound of Carolina clay covered Sandy's body. Flowers, real and artificial, decorated her grave. Then Tricia Ann, Linda, and the other mourners retired to Sandy's parents' house for the repast.

Linda and Tricia Ann stood around the yard thinking about Sandy and about the wasted life of someone so young, so beautiful, yet so flawed. Of all the funerals Linda and Tricia Ann ever attended, Sandy's was the most emotionally raw. Tricia Ann didn't cry during the funeral, but as she kept thinking about Sandy, her tears flowed.

"My tears come after the fact," she says. Linda's eyes also welled with tears, and a red blotch covered her cheeks. She dabbed the corners of her eyes with tissue. AIDS is a shared physical, spiritual, and emotional journey between patient and social worker, patient and physician, patient and family and friends. As the two women stood awash in memories of Sandy, a man approached them.

"Can I ask you a question?" he asked, a look of concern plastered over his face. "Why you are here?" Tricia Ann looked at him. Linda looked at him. Instinctively, Tricia Ann knew what the man was searching for.

"I know what y'all do," he said. Linda didn't catch on to what the man was trying to say, so Tricia Ann intervened.

"If you know what we do and you knew Sandy, do we need to . . . ?"

"I knew Sandy well, real well," he said.

Looking at him and seeing the expression on his face, Tricia Ann was convinced his relationship with Sandy was more than casual. "I knew he was with Sandy," she told herself. "How well did you know Sandy?" she asked.

"I knew her well," he replied. "She was a good friend of mine." Looking at him, trying to decipher the expression on his face and the tenderness with which he spoke, Tricia Ann instinctively knew he had been one of Sandy's lovers.

"She was a pretty girl," he said, striving for nonchalance. He knew more than he let on, but he needed to build trust with the two women before he could open up.

"Do I need to visit you?" Tricia Ann queried.

"No, no."

"What are you trying to say?" Tricia Ann asked, as the cat-and-mouse game continued. "If you knew her well, what are you trying to say to us?" she pressed him further. Tricia Ann didn't feel like being coy. After all, too many of her neighbors were lying six feet under because not enough people spoke up and told the truth.

"I just knew her well."

"Is there something you want to tell us?" she asked. "Is there something we need to do for you?"

"What do you mean?" he asked, feigning ignorance. This game was over. She got to the point.

"Do you need to be tested?" she asked.

His response stunned her. "Whatever I have, I don't want to know." The man was married.

The two women were amazed at the looks they attracted. Everyone in Cloverdale knew Tricia Ann's role with the dying. And there was Linda, a white woman, at a black funeral. Onlookers put two and two together. If they were there, it meant Sandy had this disease, the "thang."

17

NITA

Bernitha Ann Armstrong was born on June 16, 1959, in a house on Washington Street in Clover. She lived with her grandmother, Miss Jessie; her mother, Lilly; a little sister, Dorothy; and three brothers.

The Armstrong household benefited from the stability and strength of Miss Jessie Armstrong, their Christian grandmother. She looked after the grandkids when Lilly went to work. They were largely her burden. She worried about them. She fretted over them. She ruled the Armstrong household with a firm hand. But in a way, that gave Lilly an excuse to be irresponsible. She never quite grew up. Lilly loved the liquor bottle like a baby bottle, sucking for nutrition. But liquor didn't love her. When she drank, it made her easy and loose. She tried to fill the void in a self-destructive alcoholic binge that both daughters tragically inherited.

Nita's father was a short, brown-skinned man. He and Lilly were never married. One day he packed his suitcase, boarded the bus, and headed for Baltimore, Maryland. Nita grew up like too many young black girls, abandoned by her father, who fled the oppressive South in search of elusive dreams up North.

After Nita's father left, her mother sought solace in the arms of other men. Lilly brought men into the house when Nita and Dorothy were little girls. Many nights her daughters placed pillows over their ears to muffle the sounds of their mother's sexual exploits.

Dorothy and Nita feared the nights but loved the days when they could skip and play with Tricia Ann, their cousin from down the street. The three girls were bound by more than just geography. Their common poverty and blood created a strong bond among the trio. Tricia Ann's grandmother was the sister of Dorothy and Nita's grandmother, Jessie Armstrong, whom Tricia Ann called Aunt Jessie. Nita and Tricia Ann were born less than three months apart.

Although they were third cousins, Tricia Ann, Nita, and Dorothy were as close as sisters. They played hopscotch and hide-and-seek between the old run-down houses that ringed Roosevelt Park in Clover's Cloverdale neighborhood. Dorothy, the younger sibling, tagged along but was usually the odd one out.

Suddenly, Lilly got married, and she and her girls packed their suitcases and left Clover. For a few years they were just gone, as if they had never existed. Then, without notice, they reappeared. Tricia Ann returned home from school one day to find Nita and Dorothy standing in her front yard as if nothing had changed.

Tricia Ann and her cousins rekindled their friendship. On midweek nights, Tricia Ann and Dorothy walked to prayer meetings and song services. They felt protected inside the church walls. But Nita was different. Like Carolyn, she rebelled early on. She preferred the music and rhythm of the streets. She felt at home among the men and women on the street corners. Whenever they passed her on the streets, Tricia Ann and Dorothy teased her. She was too fast, flitting from the arms of one boy to the next.

As a teenager, Nita was petite and slim. Her gift was her round face, accented by dimples and an I-can-do-anything smile. A faded color photograph from the early 1970s shows her smiling, mischievous and gleeful, as she leaned against a sports car. The virus of delinquency that infected Nita must have been contagious. Within a few years, Dorothy began to skip church. The lure of the juke joints pulled her away. Maybe it was inevitable, fated by flawed genes passed down by her mother. But Dorothy soon turned to the bottle, while Tricia Ann, under the strong influence of her staunchly religious mother, made the lonely walk to church. Years later, when she encountered Dorothy on the street, the girlhood friends reminisced.

"You made the best choice," Dorothy told Tricia Ann, who by then had married Larry, given birth to four sons, and become a preacher.

"It's not too late," said Tricia Ann. But by all appearances, it might have been too late for Dorothy and her older sister. All of Dorothy's children had different fathers. Everyone in the neighborhood knew. Dorothy didn't hide anything. Liquor loosened her tongue and her morals. One day, while she was having an affair with a neighbor, Dorothy walked along the street as her married lover sat on his front porch with his wife. She brazenly propositioned him. "Terry, meet me in an hour," she said. "I'm in heat, and you can come get me."

A loud argument ensued between Dorothy and the man's wife, who knew better than to get in Dorothy's face. Dorothy was a fighter; she fought like a man. Folks on the streets of Cloverdale were afraid to mess with her.

But alcoholism was a disease Dorothy couldn't cure. She drank herself to death. She was twenty-eight. When she died in 1989, her daughter Jessie was three years old, too young to understand the shame Dorothy inflicted on the family. Jessie and her sister moved in with their grandmother. But death soon returned to the Washington Street house. After their grandmother died in 1992, Dorothy's children became wards of the state and were sent to live with foster parents.

By then, Nita, the children's closest relative, was in no shape to take in her nieces and nephew. After all, her children spent time in foster care too. For years Nita lived as a wild child, flitting along the streets and alleys, men nipping at her heels, trying to catch the butterfly. Whenever Tricia Ann encountered her on the street, Nita's breath reeked of stale beer and wine. Her eyes, once eager and white, turned bloodshot, sinister. She had fallen hard for the bottle and harder still for Dick McKee, a handsome, light-skinned mama's boy who was blessed with good hair, something that black girls everywhere found irresistible.

Everyone told Nita that Dick was crazy, but nothing would change her mind. She justified everything he did. They fought constantly. He tossed her from his moving car as he sped through Clover. When the police found Nita battered and bruised, she refused to press charges. She insisted it was an accident, a big misunderstanding. She escaped with her life, fifty-seven stitches in her head, and a broken arm. After Nita left the hospital, she moved to Gastonia. Her address changed, but her circumstances didn't. Her boyfriend still beat her. Once he broke her ribs and her nose with an iron pipe. When the police arrived on the scene he was still beating her.

Then one day Nita disappeared again. The rumor was that she had moved to Baltimore, Maryland, to live with an old lover. She stayed away, as if Clover harbored too many bad memories. Unlike some of her neighbors and girlhood friends, Nita never came home for Christmas or Easter to show off her fine, big-city clothes and northern sophistication—until, without warning, she reappeared again, a sick, broken, bitter woman who looked more like sixty-five than thirty-five. She rented an apartment from Tricia Ann's uncle. He worried about Nita. She fell ill. The neighbors whispered.

"She has that AIDS thing," her landlord said skeptically. His concern wasn't charitable. He worried about collecting his rent. He wanted Tricia Ann to find out what was wrong with Nita. After all, she was the one who cared for people with AIDS.

Tricia Ann and Nita were former best friends divided by circumstance. While Tricia Ann remained in Clover, married, and raised four boys, Nita led a rootless existence tainted by her addiction to drugs and alcohol. She made bad choices, and life repaid her in kind. Tricia Ann's days revolved around the church; her faith, inherited from her mother, helped steer her clear of many of the pitfalls that snagged her childhood friends. Tricia Ann was delighted to be reunited with her long-lost girlfriend, so she drove over to welcome her home. She knocked and walked in. "What's wrong?" she asked Nita. Nita was not exactly glad to see her old friend. "She told me to get out of her house and never come back," Tricia Ann recalled later.

Tricia Ann opened the door and left. But she went back the next day, and the same thing happened. Nita cursed her again and told her to never step over her threshold again. As she left, Tricia Ann threatened to keep coming back until Nita told her what was wrong. And she would come back again and again, even if Nita kicked her out each time. In between the volleys of language, profane enough to turn Tricia Ann's dark face red, she urged Nita to go to the doctor. Each time, Nita refused. But help was coming from an unlikely source. Tricia Ann went to bed one night and dreamed about Nita. In her dream, fire consumed a neighbor's house. As Tricia Ann arrived on the scene, bystanders watched the flames engulf the wood-frame structure, but no one tried to rescue Nita, who was inside.

"I remember saying in the dream, 'God, show me how to get in there and get her out. I won't stand there and let her burn to death.'" Tricia Ann grabbed a blanket, wet it, and dashed into the burning building. Once inside, she called out Nita's name in the thickening smoke.

"Nita! Nita!" There was no response. Then she heard a voice say to her, "Reach down and pull her leg."

She pulled until Nita's trapped body was clear, then she threw the wet blanket over her. Then Tricia Ann woke up. Some dreams are forgettable; their memory fades with the dawn. But others play like a feature movie in our waking hours, vivid and real. Tricia Ann felt compelled to share her dream with Nita. Even though Nita did not want to listen, Tricia Ann felt she had no choice. The dream seemed soaked in symbolism. But her assignment demanded patience. Nita's brittle façade took time to crack. She still cursed Tricia Ann whenever the two crossed paths.

Weeks passed before Tricia Ann made her move. By then Nita had recovered from her latest bout with illness. She returned to the streets, bottle in hand, drunk, staggering, and still belligerent. Then, in late summer 1997, Nita staggered along Queensgate Road and saw Tricia Ann standing on her front step. Reflexively, Nita's lips turned downward with an intoxicated smirk, her slurred words smeared with disdain. Tricia Ann beckoned to her.

"Come," she said. Surprise stopped Nita in her tracks.

"You want me to come in there?" she replied defiantly. "I ain't coming in. I got a beer in my hand. You wouldn't let me drink my beer." Tricia Ann let her drunken rant go unanswered for a moment, as if buying time to summon the resolve to unload the burden she had been carrying for weeks.

"Nita, I had a dream," she said, and she began to recall the troubling dream that she could not forget. As Tricia Ann retold the dream, Nita burst out laughing. She laughed long and loud as if her soul had just discovered a fountain of joy beneath the torrents of booze and bad memories.

"You gonna be my savior, to rescue me from the fiery pits of hell!"

"You're right."

Nita laughed again, but this time her levity seemed forced. Then her mood returned to defiance. "I don't want to hear that mess," she said and stormed off toward her house. Months later Nita was sick again, bad enough for her neighbors to call the ambulance to take her to the hospital in Charlotte. She almost didn't make it back home. But she couldn't shake Tricia Ann's dream. Nita and Dorothy and Tricia Ann were raised together. She was once saved. Whenever she saw Nita, Tricia Ann encouraged her friend to rediscover her faith.

"All you have to do is come back," she told her. At the time, Tricia Ann was assigned to lead a mission of the Fire Baptized Holiness Church in western York County. The congregation was small, mostly her neighbors, her friends, and their relatives. They had not yet rented the old white church with the steeple in York. On Sundays, they moved Tricia Ann's living room furniture to the walls and rearranged chairs to hold service. One day Nita walked in dressed for church. During the service, she sat quietly. She self-consciously clapped when the other worshipers sang. At the end of the service, Nita finally spoke up.

"I want what you got," she said, breaking down in tears. "I want what you got." The tears and the words flowed nonstop as Nita launched into a long confessional. All those months of rudeness and meanness were just an outward show, she said. Inside she was in turmoil. "Since that night you told me about that dream, that dream would not leave me," she told Tricia Ann. That day she went from Nita the drunk to Nita the saint.

Most drug addicts and alcoholics who discover faith struggle during the transition from their old lives to the new. They must thwart their old demons even as they seek new ways of filling the emotional and spiritual void inside. Nita was different. Her transformation was immediate.

"It was as if God knew Nita's time wasn't long. He performed an instant makeover," Tricia Ann says. "He changed her looks, he changed her smile." And he gave Nita a favorite song: "I'm Free."

In 1998 Tricia Ann and her True Word of God Fire Baptized congregation moved into the building vacated by Cedar Grove United Methodist Church when it merged with another congregation. As she stood at the pulpit, Tricia Ann used to look at her friend and marvel about how God had remade Nita into a new woman. Gone was the drunken, profane hag who stalked the streets with a bottle in her hand and misery in her heart. Her whole countenance was transformed. God resided in every sentence. Her words were lathered with faith and grace. Serenity and humility replaced the cloak of bitterness she once wore.

"She walked holy, she talked holy. She lived holy. She didn't worry what anyone thought." Nita took the word of God literally in a simple, childlike, unerring faith. Every Sunday morning she cooked and brought Tricia Ann a plate of food to eat after she preached her sermon. After standing on her feet preaching for an hour, Tricia Ann usually felt drained and tired. Nita took it upon herself to remedy that.

"The virtue has gone out of my pastor, and I need to feed her," Nita would say proudly. Despite the spiritual transformation in Nita, she could not escape the daily reality. She had AIDS. It was one miracle she didn't pray for. She struggled to take the medicine that would slow the deterioration of her immune system so that each common cold or upset stomach didn't become a life-threatening illness.

One source of inspiration for Nita was her two nieces, her sister Dorothy's daughters. They gave her reason to fight, to stay drug free, to live. Nita had given birth to a son and a daughter, now grown. She was far from the perfect mother. Men and liquor were two jealous lovers that interfered with motherhood. She moved between Baltimore and Clover. For a while the state of South Carolina had placed Nita's two children in foster care. The story was similar for Dorothy's two daughters and one son. Dorothy died of cirrhosis of the liver in 1989. Jessie, one of her daughters, was much too young to remember her mother. All she has are old, faded family pictures. For a while, the girls lived with their grandmother. When she died, they moved in with foster parents. They shuttled between foster families in Clover, then Greenville, South Carolina.

But Jessie was homesick. She wanted to be with her aunt Nita and her sister and her brother. She felt as if she were being punished for her mother's death. Then one day a car pulled up in front of the house where she lived in Greenville. She was going home to live with Aunt Nita in Rock Hill.

The aunt who greeted her at the door was not the same person Jessie remembered. Although she had been a little girl at the time, Jessie knew that her aunt was once addicted to drugs and alcohol. But this person who took Jessie and her sister in was different. "I could tell when I came back she was really clean," Jessie recalled years later. "She had been sober. She showed a lot of nurturing for us. She really cared. She really tried to make us happy while we were there."

Nita counseled Jessie and her sister about life and making the right choices. Each weekday, Jessie rode the bus to Rosewood Elementary, and every afternoon Aunt Nita stood at the bus stop anticipating her return.

Late Saturday nights or early Sunday mornings, Nita spent hours in the kitchen baking macaroni and cheese and preparing potato salad so dinner was ready as soon as they returned home from church. Her aunt's potato salad was special. Since her aunt's death, Jessie has not eaten anyone else's potato salad. Not even Tricia Ann's, who took her in.

After Nita was diagnosed with AIDS, Linda Ashley added Nita's name to her case file. But—unlike most of the other people who had AIDS—Nita was an unusually tough case. She insisted on living life on her own terms. And in 1998, Nita decided not to take any more of the medicines that would help her stave off AIDS-related infections. She went to the health department and told Linda of her decision. The two women argued. Nita told Linda she was anxious to go home. She felt ready to die. Her decision could have only one end result—her health would begin to deteriorate quickly.

The news upset Linda. She wanted Nita to fight. She respected Nita's right to self-determination, but nothing in her social work training, either at Winthrop University or at the University of South Carolina, had prepared Linda to see and accept an aunt and a mother's decision to give in to AIDS fatigue, to give up and die. Her client service manuals provided no answers to the questions of why someone with young children at home would choose death rather than cling to life, even if it was a life tainted by AIDS. Linda believed in her heart that if the doctors changed Nita's medications, it would revive her failing health and renew her will to live.

"You have to talk to that Nita," Linda urged Tricia Ann. "Did she tell you what she is going to do?"

"Yes, she discussed it with me," Tricia Ann replied. "Whatever she decided, I would back her."

"You can't do that," Linda said. "You need to encourage her to take the medicine."

"This is Nita's life," said Tricia Ann. "I don't know Nita's life. I don't know how she feels. I love her no matter what."

"But you're a preacher," Linda insisted.

"As a preacher I know that when it's God's time to take somebody home, there's nothing either you nor I could do about it," Tricia Ann replied calmly. "It's the decision she made. We need to stand by her. We need to let her know that it's going to be all right."

"Pat, you can't let her give up," Linda said. "She's just given up."

"Linda, we can't sit here and say we know what she's going through. We don't have AIDS."

Linda didn't give up. She tried a new tactic. "You and I know people who've been down a few times and they've come back," Linda said, struggling to hide her frustration. She was almost upset with Tricia Ann for not siding with her. "Is this a black thing again?" Linda asked.

"No, it's a Christian thing again," Tricia Ann said.

"You have to separate from being a pastor."

"Can I? I will always love you, but I must obey God," Tricia Ann said. "I'm sorry, Linda, if that's what you're expecting." That was a key moment in their relationship. Linda finally came around to appreciate, if not agree with, Tricia Ann's perspective.

AIDS, a silent, virulent, impatient killer, gives time only grudgingly. But it is not just the physical, debilitating aspects of the illness. AIDS also takes a financial toll on its victims. If you can't work, you can't afford to pay for food, rent, or medical care. Nita couldn't work. She hadn't held a steady job since she returned from up North. She struggled to survive on donations from the food bank. Linda used money from Catawba Care to help Nita pay for rent, utilities, and other household and personal expenses.

Despite her physical ailments, Nita was faithful in her church attendance. During the last six months of her life, she came whenever the doors were open. She especially loved to help with communion. Wearing a long, snow-white dress or skirt and her white gloves with a white prayer cap on her head, Nita evoked an image of a godly woman. The irony didn't escape those who knew her. A healthy Nita never looked quite as good as when she was dying.

In those final months, while she was still strong enough, Nita accompanied Tricia Ann wherever the pastor went to preach. As she and Tricia Ann drove out of town to visit other churches, Nita would lie down in the back-seat in the car. As each mile passed, the two women shared stories about a fun childhood that seemed as if it belonged to totally different people.

They enjoyed six months. Then, inevitably, Nita started down that irreversible slope toward the end. And when she did, unlike many of her former Clover neighbors with AIDS, Nita didn't suffer in secret. Her newly found faith freed her from shame and guilt. She was open about her illness. The last Sunday she attended church, she reclined on the pew. Members fetched a blanket and a pillow and made her comfortable. Nita asked Tricia Ann to tell the church members that she had AIDS.

Because of Tricia Ann's work, the congregation was familiar with AIDS. But the reality of the illness really hit home when she began to speak about Nita.

"Mother Armstrong is sick," Tricia Ann said quietly. "She's not going to be able to come back to church. But she wants you to know how much she loved you especially for accepting and embracing her even though she has AIDS. She's dying." Members just broke down and cried.

"You can cry now, but when we go to her house you can't cry," Tricia Ann admonished her church members. They asked questions. Could they get AIDS if they had hugged her or kissed her on the cheek? How long had she had AIDS? How long did she have to live? Did her nieces know? What were those marks on Nita's face? Church members didn't know the marks were lesions, Tricia Ann said. She didn't want them to treat Nita any differently, as if she were a leper.

After the service, Tricia Ann drove Nita home to Rock Hill.

"You don't have to come if you don't feel well," Tricia Ann told her. "We can bring church to you. On Wednesday, we can bring Bible study to you."

"That would be good," Nita replied.

The following Wednesday night a group of church members accompanied Tricia Ann to Nita's place. As they took turns praying on their knees, one earnest member, Faye, sought God's healing touch for Nita.

"Touch mother's body, bring her back to church," she prayed. Nita interrupted the prayer.

"Stop praying for that," she said without anger. "I don't you want you to pray that prayer. I'm ready to go home. Let me go home."

That reaction shocked the small group. After all, living is all we ever want to do. Whoever heard of a drowning person refusing a life raft? Although

Christianity espouses a glorious afterlife for those who believe, even the staunchest Christian, when sick, clings to life, hoping for a miracle. When Tricia Ann led Nita back into her bedroom, the sick woman repeated her warning. She didn't want anyone praying for God to heal her.

Faye slipped again. She couldn't quite break the habit of seeking God's intervention in times of trouble, but Nita cut her off.

"Didn't I tell you not to pray for my healing?"

In the late 1990s, people with AIDS lived from one infection to the next, each one threatening to be the last, each one requiring an emergency visit to the hospital. After a hospital stay in the fall of 1998, Nita wanted her own place. She and her nieces had lived with her adult daughter and boyfriend for a while, but she didn't want to move back in with them. At that stage of her life, Nita felt as if she needed peace and quiet. She also wanted to leave behind her old Clover neighborhood with its bad memories and make a fresh start.

Social workers found her an apartment in Rock Hill. Tricia Ann promised to visit her during the day to give her a bath and keep her company. Nita's daughter would stay with her at night.

"I want my room painted purple. I want flowers on my bedspread," she announced.

Tricia Ann summoned the men of the church to paint Nita's bedroom. She asked the women to buy Nita a comforter with flowers. The men painted her room, cleaned her carpet, and bought her a mattress set.

They called the ambulance to transport her home. But before the orderlies wheeled her out the door, Nita had one vital matter to settle. She wanted no last-minute delays on her trip to Glory. If she was going home, she didn't want some overzealous nurse or doctor trying to revive her. So she asked her physician to help her fill out an end-of-life designation form. "Do Not Resuscitate." Her request fulfilled, she let them wheel her to the ambulance for the drive south across the state line.

A few days after she returned home, Nita called Tricia Ann and asked her to come back to Rock Hill.

"What do you want?" Tricia Ann asked. Nita told her she had a check to cash.

"Baby, the bank is closed. We'll deal with it tomorrow."

"I will just put it under the mattress," Nita said.

"I'll be there tomorrow."

The next day she put Nita in the car, and they drove to Nita's bank. Nita cashed the check and opened a savings account. She deposited some of the money and kept some cash.

"Nita, you don't need to keep all that money," Tricia Ann cautioned. "That's too much cash to keep around the house."

"No, it's not. I want to take care of all my dues," Nita said. "I want to pay my dues for the year."

"You don't need to do that," Tricia Ann said.

"You won't cheat me out of my blessing," Nita insisted. "I'm paying my tithes. What are my dues for the year?" And the two women sat down and calculated the church's annual financial obligation, and Nita handed over her share of the responsibility. There was cash left over.

"You can put it on my burial."

After that day, Nita never really talked anymore. She slept continuously. Tricia Ann bathed her and urged her to eat, but she wouldn't. As death approaches, food, one of life's necessities, loses its luster.

Nita was a southern girl to the end. Even though her father had left her when she was young, she still loved him. Before she stopped talking, she asked to find her father, who was living in Baltimore. Tricia Ann knew his family, so she phoned a relative in Gastonia to pass along the news that Nita was dying. He called soon afterward and promised to be on the first plane out. He was scheduled to arrive on February 10, 1999.

On that Wednesday, Tricia Ann sat on the bed beside Nita as usual. Nita's restful slumber spelled death. Tricia Ann held Nita's hands, which were hot from a fever. Nita's breathing slowed. The fall and rise of her chest was almost imperceptible. Slowly, a stillness covered her body, feet first, then all the way to her eyelids. Then she opened her eyes, glanced around the room, and closed them one final time. Seated next to Nita, holding her hands, Tricia Ann marveled at the mystery of life and death.

"You can be right there, but if it's not your time to go you can't go," she says. "Even though my hand was in her hand, it didn't take me."

Nita was only thirty-nine.

18

MOVING ON

In 1999, the board of directors for the Close Foundation, a Charlotte-area philanthropic organization, met to consider grant applications. Among the requests was one from a new organization, the Catawba Care Coalition, seeking $80,000 in seed money to open an AIDS clinic that would serve people living with AIDS and HIV in a three-county area, including people in Clover. In the boardroom sat Tammy Whisenant, assistant to the foundation's president and the older sister of Chris Blanton, the York County AIDS Task Force ombudsman. As the deliberations began, one board member objected to the clinic's request. "We don't have AIDS here," he said. "We don't have gay people in Lancaster County."

At that time, at least 560 people in the area had been diagnosed with HIV, yet the man still dared to believe the problem belonged only to New York and San Francisco. As Tammy sat at the table listening to him, she felt as if she would explode. Here was a successful businessman and colleague who was oblivious to the problem at his doorstep.

Meanwhile, Linda Ashley was at home hoping for good news. She had staked her career on a gamble. She had left the relative security of the York County health department to launch this new venture. The recently incorporated nonprofit Catawba Care Coalition needed money to open a privately run clinic to treat people with HIV and AIDS. She had launched out in faith; she couldn't turn back. There was nothing to go back to. The time for timidity was over since the knock on her hotel door that night years before when her friends greeted her with the news of her son's suicide. Since then, she had broken one convention after the other.

After three years, Linda was tired of the health department, its limitations, its rules, and its lack of vision. People were dying of AIDS, and the bureaucrats in Columbia didn't seem to care about what happened in small places like Clover. Linda chafed at the constraints of the job and the untapped possibilities her position offered. She believed the health department had room for an HIV/AIDS clinic. It wasn't a novel idea. Bamberg County, a place without the population or resources of York County, had begun a county health department AIDS clinic seven years before Linda spoke to her first AIDS client.

For Linda, the main issue was the lack of decent medical care. Locally, social workers looked to Dr. Tracy Timony to treat AIDS patients, although she was an internist and not an infectious disease specialist. There was not one full-time infectious disease physician in the health department district that included York, Chester, and Lancaster counties. One was badly needed. At that time, in the mid-1990s, Lancaster boasted one of the highest syphilis infection rates in the country. "Folks if they were seeing a doctor were seeing Tracy," Linda said. "She was good, but she couldn't see all of them. That was the biggest gap—no infectious disease doctor."

Every day, as she worked the phones seeking better treatment options for dying men and women, her frustration grew. It seemed inconceivable that, more than fifteen years after the first people were diagnosed with what became known as AIDS, her community still lacked a physician with the skill and knowledge to treat patients with the illness.

One day, while she was walking the hallways of Piedmont Medical Center worried about a person with AIDS who was fighting for his life, Linda saw Dr. Phil Lackey striding toward her. He worked for ID Consultants, a Charlotte-based infectious disease practice. Linda didn't know it, but Phil Lackey's medical career up until that point seemed to be training for that very moment and the hard task that lay ahead. As Lackey walked down the hallway, Linda stepped into his path. The mischievous smile on her face was so big it almost knocked off her glasses.

"You are just wonderful," she said to him. "Would you consider open-ing a clinic in Rock Hill?" She wasn't talking about just an ordinary clinic. Linda wanted a clinic for people with HIV and AIDS.

"Well, I might consider it," he replied, somewhat surprised at her blunt approach. "We don't have the money. We're not a big practice."

Linda saw an opening and pounced. "If I get a clinic, would you come?" she asked.

His eyes brightened. "I'll think about it," he said. "I probably will."

"The fire was lit," Linda recalled much later. "He was a cooked goose, and he didn't know it."

What made her even more desperate to establish an AIDS clinic was the knowledge that other small towns across the state had figured out ways to meet the needs of people with AIDS and HIV. For three years she had attended meetings in Columbia and listened to others talk about offering quality medical care treatment that was not readily available to people who lived in Clover and Rock Hill. Finally, Linda had found her doctor. All she had to do now was find a place for her clinic.

The space was a vacant office near a family-owned pharmacy five min-utes from the Rock Hill city center. The owner appreciated a long-term tenant. In May 2000, the Christopher Clinic opened its doors. Dr. Lackey came by for a few hours a week to treat patients who drove from as far as Chester to the south, Lancaster to the east, and Clover to the west.

Soon afterward, Linda set about writing a federal grant application to the Ryan White program, the largest federal program designed for people living with HIV and AIDS. Since it was enacted in 1990, the legislation opened the doors for state and local governments and community-based organizations to provide medical care and support services for individuals and families afflicted by HIV and AIDS. In 1991, the federal government awarded the state of South Carolina $689,000 in Ryan White CARE Act funds to set up a network of services, which was sorely lacking at the time.

As a nonprofit community-based organization, the Catawba Care Coalition was eligible for Part C Outpatient Early Intervention Services program funds. The paperwork complete, Linda submitted the application and waited. Federal agencies announce grant awards through the local congressional office, so the member of the House of Representatives could take credit for federal largesse. News of their Ryan White grant came from a staff member in Representative John Spratt's office that spring of 2001. The agency had secured a grant for $600,000. It had hit the jackpot.

Linda was so excited about the news that she ran down the hallway and almost tripped, one staffer recalled.

With the Ryan White CARE Act money in 2001, the agency took another step. Before then they had subcontracted with another AIDS agency in Charlotte for Dr. Lackey's services at the Christopher Clinic. Now they didn't need to do that. They were able to contract directly with ID Consultants for Dr. Lackey's services.

While the infectious disease specialist provided primary outpatient care for those with HIV and AIDS, the grant allowed the Christopher Clinic's four staff members to provide HIV counseling and other health services to low-income and medically underserved people living with HIV/AIDS.

Health Resources and Services Administration records show that after the initial $600,000, the Catawba Care Coalition received other grants, including a much smaller check for $120,000 the following year. Then in 2003, the grant rose to $446,240 and $400,000 for two consecutive years, 2004 and 2005. Coupled with Housing Opportunities for People with AIDS grants from the US Department of Housing and Urban Development and money from private foundations, the Christopher Clinic was on firm financial footing. Linda had tried to hire nurse Faye Ballard away from the county health department when she first opened the clinic. Eventually, Ballard did leave the relative security of her state job to work at the clinic.

During the early years, the clinic focused on supportive services—buying food, finding AIDS patients an apartment, and supplying rides back and forth to the clinic. Caseworkers did everything for their clients. They took them grocery shopping, helped with their rent, got them telephone service, scheduled their medical appointments, and ensured they kept them.

"We were helping people die," said Anita Case, whom Linda hired in 2001 to serve as the agency's supervisor for case management. Case had studied sociology and religion at Wake Forest University and obtained a master's degree in social work at the University of North Carolina at Chapel Hill. She stayed at Catawba Care Coalition for three years before leaving for an agency in Florence.

During her years at the county health department and the Christopher Clinic, Linda encountered people of every sort. They came black, white, gay, and straight, men and women, even transsexuals. They shared one common condition: AIDS.

Many of those visitors to Linda's office sat in her wooden rocker and wrapped themselves with an afghan she had knitted when she was a young girl. Often they sat and rocked back and forth, hugging the blanket as they talked and cried. "They felt so good and so safe," said Margaret Jenkins.

"It was not just a doctor's office," added Tricia Ann. "It was a place where you could go and find peace and serenity and know it was OK."

The names and faces of those visitors occupy a place in Linda's memory like the countless baby pictures in a pediatrician's office. She remembers the lessons they taught her, the conversations they had. But none stand out like Eugene. Social workers spend their days trying to help the worst and least among us. After a while, though, cynicism creeps in, and they come only to expect the worst. Eugene, an ex-convict, helped Linda see her own prejudices. "Eugene taught me a lesson," she says. "When you're a social worker, you work hard at being nonjudgmental."

But she struggled to get past her feelings about people who spent time behind bars. Eugene served ten years in prison for burglary of a store. When Linda first heard about him, she visualized a tough, rough-looking man. But into her office walked a slight gentleman dressed in a suit and tie. "I am sitting there thinking, have I got the right person here?" she said years later.

Like so many young black men, Eugene got in trouble by hanging around with the wrong crowd. One night they went out drinking and then robbed a store. But Eugene and his friends were too drunk to realize that the burglar alarm had gone off. Police caught them in the act. By the time he was released from state prison a decade later, Eugene had the symptoms of full-blown AIDS. He moved in with his mother and stepfather, but they treated him like a leper. He was confined to a back room and made to use paper plates and plastic forks. Each time he used the bathroom, his mother came behind him to clean up with bleach.

Since Eugene was a convicted felon, US Department of Housing and Urban Development rules barred him from public housing. So the Rock Hill Housing Authority, which received federal money, refused to allow Eugene to live in one of the city's public apartments. The Catawba Care Coalition appealed. But the housing director was a one-man appeal board. He sat at the end of the table with his arms folded. At the end of the hearing, he was noncommittal. "You will be notified in two weeks' time," he said.

"He wouldn't even tell us what the decision might be," Linda says. "I knew I could not change his mind."

He rejected Eugene's application. In desperation, Linda appealed to the public housing director in a nearby town. She explained Eugene's unusual circumstances, which required a different approach. Eugene's case led to the formation of the AIDS Housing Coalition. "I could have gone to the Rock Hill guy and slapped him in his face," she says. "It didn't matter. He didn't care."

Eugene was one of her less tragic cases. After another of Linda's AIDS clients died, Eugene married the man's widow. Several years later he too succumbed to the disease. He was only about fifty.

Did southern black and white folk, men and women, react differently to having AIDS? Almost everyone broke down. The news plunged them into depression; some even considered suicide. Women were more open about disclosing how they got infected, Linda found. "Men lied a lot."

The guys, both white and black, unless they were openly gay, never wanted to admit they'd had any kind of homosexual relations or that they had had sex with a prostitute. And men were more apt to lie about how many sexual partners they'd had. Women were usually so devastated about being infected that they didn't care about hiding. They were so mad they usually wanted to kill whoever had infected them.

The biggest difference across the races, black and white, Linda learned over the years, was in the degree of denial. Among blacks the wall of silence was almost absolute. "You weren't allowed to talk about it at all," Linda says.

Among whites, infected men and women were more likely to admit they were HIV positive and risk rejection. But for African Americans, the stigma seeped deep into their cultural marrow. The double stigma of being gay and HIV positive stung terribly. It led to denial, which doctors found usually led to early death. Some came home from up North back to their rural hometowns like Clover with deception and illness. In fleeing the cities, they left behind their support systems, their lifelong friends, to come home to the social and cultural isolation of being gay in a conservative southern town.

"They expect their family to take care of them thinking they had cancer and knowing all along it was HIV," Linda said. "Do you choose to be true to yourself, or do you choose to come home and be close to your family? They usually live a lie."

One day a man walked through the door. He was a minister. His T cell count was seventeen. Linda had never seen anyone with a T cell count that low. The man had had HIV for a long time, and it had progressed to AIDS. He knew but was unwilling to take the chance of anyone else finding out. He was not about to be caught dead going to an AIDS clinic. He ended up in the hospital.

Then there was the married minister who wouldn't come to the clinic if any other clients were around. He scheduled his visits early in the morning or late in the afternoon or pretended he was there for something other than medical care. Sometimes Linda would meet him in a church or another office so nobody would suspect the truth. He was bisexual. He refused to talk about how he was infected. "That's a tough way to live and an even tougher way to die," she says. The minister didn't live long. "That level of denial will kill you."

AIDS also brought out the best in some people. "I have had more than a few people say to me, 'AIDS was the best thing that happened to me,'" she recalls. "It said to them, 'Get your life straight, now.' Not physically but in terms of finding peace."

Folks who had never before looked for healthy, peaceful places inside themselves worked desperately to find them when they fell ill. However, others, such as one Clover man, Jim, became resentful and mean. Jim was a fifty-something, short, little man who, Tricia Ann later learned, may have been infected by having sex with Sandy, one of the early AIDS cases in Clover. "He loved him some Sandy," Tricia Ann says.

But Jim was also one of the most hateful and bitter AIDS patients Linda and Tricia Ann ever encountered. When he learned he was HIV positive, all hell broke loose. When Linda sent caseworkers to his house, they often returned in tears. Finally, Linda visited Jim.

"If you don't straighten up, nobody is going to come see you," she told him.

"You go on, Linda," he replied nonchalantly.

Soon afterward, Jim called Tricia Ann. "I'm hungry. I want some chicken and rice." Tricia Ann had just returned home from work, but she dropped everything and prepared the food and delivered it to Jim. He took it out of her hand, removed the cover, looked at it, and then tossed the food into the trash bin.

"I wanted fried chicken," he said. At that moment, Tricia Ann felt like reaching down and pushing Jim out of his wheelchair. She vowed never to set foot in his house again.

"That was my food. Next time you're hungry, don't call my house."

Fighting AIDS requires having the right attitude and taking the right medication. Jim did neither. Finally, he got so sick he needed hospice care. But he chased away every nurse. One day near the end, as a nurse walked into the house, Jim was in an especially sour mood. "If you come near me I am going to bite you and you are going to get AIDS," he threatened.

"He was a bitter little old man," Linda said. "His attitude: 'I am dying, and I am going to control what I can control.'"

19

DR. PHIL LACKEY

Phil Lackey was a tall, slim man with the kind of smile that put even the sickest patient at ease. He moved with a nonchalance that belied his intensity. He was born in Greensboro but moved to Winston-Salem with his parents when he was six years old. Phil grew up comfortably middle class with his patent attorney father, his stay-at-home mother, and a younger brother.

Lackey didn't need much convincing to work with people who were afflicted by AIDS. The University of North Carolina School of Medicine graduate had first encountered the disease during his internship at the University of Alabama–Birmingham medical school. When he first arrived in Birmingham, Lackey wanted to be an internist. But at medical school, all his favorite professors were infectious disease specialists. One, Dr. Michael Saag, really impressed him. When he was a first-year intern, Lackey also met Craig Charles, then a senior resident at UAB. The fight against HIV and AIDS would reunite the two physicians years later.

As part of his training, Lackey worked long hours at the UAB 1917 Clinic, which was one of the first full-service clinics in the Deep South to treat people with HIV and AIDS. While serving as a second-year fellow at the clinic, he met Danny Aulds, a twenty-eight-year-old whose life story was later told by his wife, Karen, in a book, *My Grace Is Sufficient: A Story of God's Grace in the Midst of AIDS*.

When he was a teenager, Danny had contracted hepatitis, then AIDS, from blood transfusions while being treated for injuries suffered in a forklift accident at a lumber mill. After he was diagnosed, Danny sought his pastor for counseling. "He went to his minister, who told him, 'God is punishing you for something you did,'" Lackey said.

Danny disagreed. He told his pastor, "That's not right."

"He spent the rest of his life speaking to church groups telling them that this is not some wrath of God," Lackey recalled. By the time Lackey met him, Danny's days of speechmaking were long over. Danny remained cheerful even as he faced death. He had every bad complication with HIV. In the end, he was infected with PML—progressive multifocal leukoencephalitis, a viral illness physicians rarely see any more, even in people with AIDS.

The day before he died, Danny asked his wife to type a letter that Lackey still keeps in his office. "Don't worry about me," he wrote. "I know I am going to be OK."

With his formal training complete, Lackey returned to his home state and began practicing medicine in Goldsboro, a town of less than forty thousand, including the military personnel at nearby Seymour Johnson Air Force Base. But after the intensity of the 1917 Clinic in Birmingham, the two years he spent in Goldsboro must have felt like a season in medical purgatory.

"You want to go where you're needed," Lackey says. And Goldsboro didn't have the population to occupy a full-time infectious disease specialist, so Lackey ended up treating maladies internists usually deal with. His passion lay elsewhere. "I wanted to do infectious diseases," he says.

When Linda accosted Lackey in the hospital hallway, he worked for ID Consultants in Charlotte on the other side of the state line. Although York County had more than a hundred thousand residents, it lacked a full-time infectious disease specialist. People with HIV often had their friends or relatives drive them thirty miles north to the big city for anonymity and care at ID Consultants or other doctors' offices.

Before Lackey could accept Linda's offer, he had to convince his medical partners that they could let him go for half a day per week. Linda's role was to negotiate how much to pay him. "I finally convinced them that it would make money for them in the long run, seeing all those people from South Carolina who didn't have any money," she says.

After much looking, Linda had found an empty office building near a pharmacy within walking distance of the Winthrop University campus. The property shared parking with several other businesses, so people with AIDS could come and go without worrying about being noticed. In May 2000, the nonprofit Catawba Care Coalition opened the Christopher Clinic, named in honor of Chris Blanton for his pioneering work as the local AIDS ombudsman.

That fall I spoke to Dr. Lackey for the first time. As the clinic's infectious disease physician, Lackey had treated Jackie, one of about thirty of Tricia Ann's Cloverdale neighbors living with AIDS.

At the time, Jackie weighed about eighty-five pounds. A cyst from AIDS blinded her left eye. Disease and hard living had ravaged her teeth and gums. Jackie was twenty-nine, but her lean face looked as if it belonged to a sixty-five-year-old woman. HIV/AIDS is a battle between a patient's viral load and her T cell counts. As the illness progresses, the viral load climbs while the T cell counts drop. Jackie's T cell count was zero. Her body was defenseless against the countless opportunistic infections that would rage in her thin frame. "Her viral load completely covers her body," Tricia Ann told me back then.

At the time, as November turned into December, Jackie's eyes were fixed not on her illness but on Christmas. She wanted to fulfill her children's wishes for the holidays. She promised Tricia Ann and Dr. Lackey that she would tell her children about her illness after the holidays. She delayed, however, hoping that if she took her meds, her condition would improve. But Jackie's condition was worse than the young woman was willing to admit. I met Jackie on Tuesday. On Wednesday she visited Dr. Lackey at the Christopher Clinic. He decided to stop Jackie's AIDS medication.

"She is not responding to the medicine," Lackey said. "She wasn't able to enjoy what time she had left. Some patients are going toward the end of life, and there is not much you can do."

Jackie died several months later. Tricia Ann buried six neighbors who had been AIDS patients in 1999, and four in 2000. Jackie was one of about half a dozen AIDS deaths in 2001. The deaths would mount with the years.

"It's very much a public health concern," said Lackey, who at the time suspected that there were many more people walking around with undiagnosed and untreated HIV.

"The scary thing is these are the ones we know about," he said. "It's only the tip of the iceberg."

While there were a number of whites with HIV/AIDS in Clover, the majority of the infected people were black. The son of a prominent white family committed suicide under the weight of the ostracism he received after being diagnosed with HIV. African Americans were being hit harder with HIV/AIDS than any other group in South Carolina, accounting for 67 percent of the 15,872 HIV cases reported through March 2000, according to the state Department of Health and Environmental Control. Adults ages twenty to forty-four were the hardest hit group. The highest HIV/AIDS infection rates occurred in the state's rural counties of Jasper, McCormick, Marlboro, Allendale, and Bamberg, where Dr. Michael Watson operated the county AIDS clinic.

As the medical director for the Christopher Clinic, Lackey saw seventy-three patients. Some area residents who could afford to visited Lackey at his ID Consultants practice in Charlotte. When they became deathly ill, they preferred to be admitted to hospitals in Charlotte and Gastonia, North Carolina. Their cases were not included in South Carolina's HIV/AIDS reports. They became a part of North Carolina's death toll for AIDS.

"It's a much bigger problem in York County than the community at large believes," Lackey said in 2000. The more rural the setting, the more outdated the beliefs. "People still think it's a gay disease," Lackey said. "They don't realize they can get it by having heterosexual sex."

Lackey worked part time at the Christopher Clinic for two years before his ID Consultants practice got so busy he had to quit. "He came to say he wasn't going to be around anymore," Linda recalled. But Lackey didn't come empty-handed. He recommended his replacement, Dr. Craig Charles, a fellow University of North Carolina medical school graduate, who was coming to work at Piedmont Medical Center. "He's a great guy," Lackey told Linda. "I want you to meet him and interview him."

"I liked him," Linda recalls. "I thought he'd fit." Still, she had some misgivings. "My fear was he would up and have a private practice," Linda says. But he didn't want to do that. Dr. Charles wanted to do hospital work. "It was the perfect match for us."

20

DR. CRAIG CHARLES

Craig Charles grew up in the furniture-manufacturing hub of Lexington, North Carolina. His father worked as an industrial welder while his mother stayed at home. Craig's father died when Craig was thirteen, and his mother went to work as an operator with the locally owned telephone company in Lexington. She never remarried.

In high school, Craig's buddies talked incessantly about going to UNC–G, the University of North Carolina at Greensboro. Craig liked the idea. The school wasn't prestigious like UNC–Chapel Hill, Duke, or Wake Forest, but he'd follow his older sister, who was the first person in his immediate family to attend college. Years later, he earned his MD a week after she got her master's degree in education.

After graduation, Craig and several high school friends drove to Greensboro. It was far enough from home for them to enjoy the experience of being independent for the first time but close enough to get home quickly if the need arose. The buddies roomed together. Craig's major was biology. When friends scoffed at what he would do with his science degree, Craig always had his answer ready.

Although UNC–Greensboro was a relatively small university, the faculty knew how to prep students for medical school. Scores of students used UNC–G as a gateway for Wake Forest, East Carolina, and even Duke University medical school. Craig opted for the University of North Carolina–Chapel Hill, the crown jewel of the Tar Heel university system. Many of his med school classmates had come from more prestigious private and state schools—Duke, Wake Forest, Clemson, Davidson.

In medical school, Craig Charles was two years ahead of Phil Lackey. The two never met in Chapel Hill. It was not until Dr. Charles was a resident at the UAB hospital that he first met Dr. Lackey. Charles was a senior resident, while Lackey was a first-year intern on service. They worked together for a month in Birmingham. "I was his boss," Charles says. "I always joked that I taught Phil."

While Lackey remained in Birmingham an extra three years to complete an infectious disease fellowship, Charles toiled in Brundidge, a small town in southeast Alabama, to fulfill his National Health Service Corps obligation. That was his way of repaying the US government for financing his med school education. As part of that program, newly minted physicians work for a set number of years in economically depressed, medically underserved areas of the country. And Brundidge was in pretty bad shape. At the time, the town had lost its main industry when the textile mills closed. Hundreds of people were unemployed, uninsured, and down-on-their-luck poor.

Early in his three-year stay in Brundidge, Dr. Charles realized he didn't want to be an internist. "It was a very difficult place to practice," he says. "I was the only doctor in town." That was the longest three years of his life. But as his time in Brundidge was coming to an end, Dr. Charles longed for something more challenging than general practice. He talked to his wife, Martha, about returning to school for a fellowship in infectious disease. Like Lackey, Dr. Charles had been impressed and inspired by his instructors in Birmingham.

During his first rotation a week after he arrived in Birmingham for his internship, Dr. Charles had been assigned to work with Dr. Bill Dismukes, then chief of infectious diseases at the university hospital. He spent a week alongside Dr. Dismukes and the rest of the month with another legend, Dr. Michael Saag.

Later, as he was preparing to leave Brundidge, Dr. Charles turned on the TV one morning to see Dr. Saag being interviewed on NBC's *Today* show. He took that as a sign he had made the right decision. "We were giddy," he said of himself and Martha. "We were going back to civilization."

For his fellowship, Dr. Charles returned to North Carolina and enrolled at Wake Forest Baptist Hospital, a facility known for its research. But he had no intention of spending his hours isolated in a research lab. "I'm a doer," he says. "I enjoy taking care of people."

After he completed his infectious disease fellowship in 1996, Dr. Charles signed a five-year deal with a private practice in Winston-Salem. For a while, it looked as if this would be the place he would work for the rest of his life.

But the same urge that pushes men and women to test their wits against strange new infectious diseases also pushes them to take on other new challenges. As he approached the end of his contract, Dr. Charles put out feelers in search of new opportunities. He wrote to medical practices in Raleigh and Greensboro, but no one responded. Then one day at work, his pager vibrated. Routinely, a page means that a patient needs care. That day it was a call from a recruiter in Texas.

"Do you know where Rock Hill, South Carolina, is?" the recruiter asked. "Would you be interested in working at a hospital there?" Charles promised to think about it, but his wife wasn't too impressed. She was from Alabama. At the time the couple had two boys and was expecting a third child. "We came down and met everyone and looked around," he says. His employers made it easier for him to leave. They wanted him to do more general practice and less infectious disease medicine.

"At that time the practice said, 'We probably need you to do more of this and less of that,'" he recalled. Dr. Charles wanted to do the opposite. With AIDS raging and destroying the lives of many of his patients, Dr. Charles wanted to focus more, not less, on infectious diseases. After all, infectious disease is a demanding field. "It's a complicated field of study," he says. "If you don't do a lot you get rusty. If you take care of diabetes and hypertension and don't spend a lot of time on infectious diseases you end up becoming poor on both."

Linda Ashley called Dr. Charles to talk about the clinic before he left Winston-Salem. He liked what he heard. Although Dr. Charles hadn't moved to Rock Hill, in his mind he had already accepted the position to be the medical director at the Christopher Clinic.

"It just worked out. I was stepping into a situation, like a perfectly fitting pair of shoes." Dr. Charles worked full time at Piedmont Medical Center, where he was the infectious disease consultant. Twice a week, he drove less than five minutes from the hospital to the Christopher Clinic. He saw HIV and AIDS patients six hours a week, on Tuesday afternoons and Thursday mornings. A full-time nurse practitioner, who could write prescriptions, worked Monday through Friday.

On average, Dr. Charles saw about a dozen returning patients and one or two new patients a week at the clinic. That's where he first saw Carolyn. She was one of his more memorable cases, not because of anything she did but because, unlike many other patients, Carolyn had a sister who fought harder for her than she did for herself.

Dr. Charles also recalls the patient who was brought in by a neighbor. He had no family members but was lucky enough to have a neighbor who checked on him. He was HIV positive and in pretty bad shape. The minute the patient walked into Dr. Charles's consulting room at the Christopher Clinic, the physician sensed this case was unsalvageable. Still he tried to be upbeat. "We are going to do what we can," he told the fifty-something man.

His intellect told him otherwise. He felt it was too late. "We may do everything right and everything may still go wrong," he says. "This was a person who was coming to us way too late." The man died two days later.

One of Dr. Charles's favorite patients was the man he met a week after he arrived in Rock Hill. Kaposi's sarcoma covered the patient's skin. Bluish blotches smeared his chest and his face and closed one eye. "He looked like a poster child for the worse case of AIDS you can imagine." Dr. Charles prescribed new medicine for the man. He was a good patient. He took his meds regularly. A year later, all of the tumors had vanished and the man looked like a regular guy on the street. He lived almost a decade longer.

"For years he was my success story," Charles says.

Eventually though, that patient died, just like too many of the men and women Charles loved and cared for.

21

CAROLYN:
THE FINAL YEARS

Two days after Sandy's pink-robed body and carnations were laid to rest, a pall of loss still hung over much of Cloverdale. But one person, Carolyn, had reason to celebrate. On October 8, 1998, her parole ended. She no longer needed to check in with her parole officer. She had served her time; now she was physically and legally free. The burning question for all who knew her was, could she keep her nose clean and stay out of prison? The answer wasn't obvious. After she left prison, Carolyn went wild. She did anything to get drugs, and somehow she managed to stay out of prison.

But Carolyn didn't stay out of trouble because she became a girl scout. She was clever enough not to prey on any more white women. She preyed on those who loved her most—her family. She stole the cash her sister brought home from her congregation's collection plate. One Sunday as Tricia Ann returned home from church, she saw a woman sitting on a front porch. The woman waved at Tricia Ann, who noticed she was wearing a floral dress similar to one Tricia Ann had recently bought on sale at a Belk's department store. But she had never worn it. As the woman passed out of sight, Tricia Ann mentioned it to Larry.

"She's got a dress just like mine," she said. When they reached home, Tricia Ann walked into the bedroom closet to compare her dress with the one she had just seen. The hanger where it once hung sat as naked as a branch without leaves. She knew immediately. Carolyn had stolen her dress and sold it to this girl, she thought. Her calmness from the Sunday service dissipated like water from a kitchen sink. Tricia Ann stormed up the street to confront the woman. She went straight to the point. "Carolyn sold you this dress?" she asked. Yes, she had.

That was one of the few occasions when stolen merchandise resurfaced. Typically, Tricia Ann and her husband left home and returned to discover their refrigerator or freezer emptier than when they left. Large cuts of steaks and freezer bags with seasoned chicken had taken wing. Carolyn stole anything that had a price tag and sold the stolen merchandise to get money to pay for her drug habit. After the incident with the dress, Tricia Ann couldn't take it anymore. She had to put her sister out.

"As hard as it was, she was tearing my house apart," Tricia Ann says. She issued Carolyn an ultimatum: get help or get out. Tricia Ann then called Linda Ashley to get help for her sister, but by the time Linda arrived, Carolyn had changed her mind. She wasn't going to get help; she wasn't getting out. "I put her out."

As a compromise, Linda drove Carolyn to Keystone, a Rock Hill inpatient rehab center. As Carolyn sat in the processing room answering questions from the social worker, Linda overheard the conversation.

"How often do you do drugs?"

"What kind of drugs?"

The answers didn't surprise Linda, but it must have pained her to hear Carolyn detail her self-destruction in an unemotional, almost clinical tone. Then the social worker asked Carolyn how much she spent daily on drugs.

"Three hundred dollars," Carolyn replied, as if she was admitting to eating cold cereal for breakfast every day. Linda almost fell out of her seat. Her mouth dropped open with disbelief. Linda spent many days worrying about finding money for groceries for Carolyn only to hear her talk about spending a week's wages on drugs every single day. Soon afterward, Carolyn checked in, and Linda left. Four weeks later, Carolyn checked herself out and left drug rehab for the streets.

Carolyn was adept at staying out of jail, but would she stay healthy?

Soon after Carolyn left rehab, the Catawba Care Coalition helped her move into her first decent apartment in York, the county seat about half an hour's ride from her old Cloverdale neighborhood. Tricia Ann and Linda hoped that removing Carolyn from her old Clover and Gastonia friends would create a safe enough distance for her to finally kick her habit and become the kind of mother she always spoke of trying to become. I visited Carolyn in that apartment in November 2000. I planned to write a series of newspaper columns to coincide with World AIDS Day that year. I hadn't seen her in a while. When she opened the door, she was dressed like a suburban housewife in a dark-colored sweat suit; her hair was short, straightened, and neatly styled. Her face was pockmarked with acne, but her high cheekbones stood out. She looked attractive, the kind of black woman who despite her heavyset build would always get a second look from a man on the street.

Her second-floor apartment was nicely furnished; a dark-colored couch and love seat framed a glass-covered cocktail table. The apartment was dimly lit except for the flickering red and orange flame of the scented candles that sat on the cocktail table. In one corner, a television game show entertained no one as Carolyn talked to me about what it meant to have AIDS. I didn't know then that this period of stability was just a respite before another reckless, suicidal binge of drugs and sex. But at that moment, after years of not taking her medicines, she was trying to be a good patient. It was hard for her. Her medications made her feel sick. Weeks earlier she had stopped taking the medication that protected her against the onslaught of opportunistic infections that could overwhelm her compromised immune system like sandbars before a hurricane. Whenever she swallowed the pills, they made her vomit constantly. She'd stoop over the toilet, heaving until there was nothing left inside her stomach, as if AIDS had stolen everything and was demanding more. She was lethargic and listless. She couldn't think straight. Her head hurt. Cramps assaulted her abdomen like period pains.

"All I could do was get up and take a dose and lay back down," she said. As she spoke, she sat listlessly on the couch. Light from the television screen mingled with the flames from her scented candles. "I have good days and bad days," she said between trips to the bathroom. "When I feel sick I just lay around."

At the time, Carolyn wanted me to call her by the pseudonym "Lynn." Although she spoke about her illness to small groups around town, and her sister spoke widely about Carolyn's plight, Carolyn was still uncomfortable letting the whole world know she had AIDS. But whenever she was invited to talk and she had the strength and courage to speak up, Carolyn always warned the young men and women about the dangers of unprotected sex. It was her way of trying to help somebody. This was not a sentiment she expressed often. "If I can get one person to listen," she said. "I would prefer abstinence, but if you have sex, for God's sake get a condom."

As I sat on the couch and listened to her, Carolyn words were filled with regret. Hers was the self-recrimination that wracks a mother who is dying of a preventable disease. "I have to keep it real with you. Drugging and unprotected sex is not cool," she told me. "Whatever it took to get drugs, I did. Look at what it cost me. I look healthy, but not a day passes without feeling the pain.

"No matter how many times I tried to blame somebody else, it always came back to me. I knew about AIDS, but when you are doing drugs, you don't care."

Her decision to stop taking her meds created a dilemma, a conflict of the two emotions that dominated her life as AIDS patient and mother: her sense of well-being and her love for her son. Some might have considered her decision selfish, just like the way she lived her entire life, just for Carolyn, for herself, for the moment. Carolyn didn't take the medicine because it made her feel sick. As long as she didn't take her medication, she felt energetic enough to take her son to the neighborhood park and play after school. She could think clearly enough to help him with his arithmetic homework and reading assignments. Because of all the moves between his aunt's house and his nomadic mother, Carolyn's son, Tremaine, was behind in school. He struggled with reading and writing. Carolyn, the former junior high school dropout, had no big dreams for her son finishing at the top of his class. She came from a family of dropouts; few if any of her siblings had earned a high school diploma. Carolyn just wanted her son to graduate from high school. And more than anything, she wanted to stand in the auditorium and cheer him as his name was called and he walked across the stage. He did; she didn't.

That day in the fall of 2000, we talked about the conflict of present feelings and future desires. Was it better for her to live longer and have more time with her son even if that time was spent in pain and discomfort? It was the kind of choice no mother should be asked to make. But it was no accident. She was not a victim. Her actions had placed her in the untenable position of having to choose either present fun or future absence. "He is the only reason why I haven't given up," she said. "He's my world."

She was thirty-six at the time, middle age for her notoriously short-living family. "My special prayer is to be able to see my son take care of himself," she said. "If God gives me that, I think I can die in peace."

People who begin treatment soon after they are diagnosed with the human immunodeficiency virus can survive for decades. But Carolyn was not one of those. Could she hold on, despite the odds, for eight more years?

All the signs suggested the answer was no. A week after we talked about her decision to abandon her drug regimen, an ugly rash, likely AIDS-related lesions, appeared on Carolyn's arms, face, and legs. In a panic, she went to her physician, Dr. Lackey, the infectious disease specialist at the Christopher Clinic, who convinced her to return to her medication. This was familiar territory for Dr. Lackey, who treated numerous patients who had endured long enough to go through AZT and hang on until the new, more effective protease inhibitors were prescribed.

"We have enough medications where we can find one that can fit and you don't feel bad," Lackey told me at the time.

In early 2001, Tricia Ann had retained full custody of her nephew, but she allowed Tre to spend more and more time with his mother so the two could finally bond. Carolyn seemed anxious, almost desperate, to make a life for them both. She spent hours of the day looking forward to the time when her son returned home from school. That was a brief period of optimism, a moment of respite, for those who best knew Carolyn. It was the happiest and most content period in her life.

"I knew how much she loved him," Tricia Ann says. "I thought him being there would settle her down." But relapse and resolve interchanged and intersected throughout Carolyn's adult life. She'd make dramatic pronouncements about kicking her habit. By 2001, she could no longer fool herself about her chances of long-term survival. Despite promises to the contrary, she never quite won the battle against addiction. Whenever she grew frustrated, her default position was to go out and get high. Sometimes when Tricia Ann visited her sister, she could sense that the agitation and the old cravings were about to return. Then she knew it was time to put distance between Carolyn and her son.

"She would have spells when she got sick and she wanted to die," Tricia Ann says. When she backslid and returned to heroin, Carolyn decided to give up the apartment. She wanted to return to New Jersey to live with her brother William. And she needed money. So Carolyn got yard sale signs and posted them around her apartment complex. That Saturday she held her first and only yard sale. The merchandise consisted mainly of furniture—the bed, the couch, loveseats, mirrors. She sold it all. At the end of the day, Carolyn showed off the wad of cash. The money was not for her usual drugs. It was to pay for her trip north. There was only one problem with her plan. The furniture wasn't hers—it was rented.

After Carolyn sold the furniture, moved out of the apartment, and relocated to New Jersey, the local furniture rental office staff pulled up in front of Tricia Ann's house in Clover. The men were looking for Carolyn and their furniture.

Before Carolyn boarded the bus for New Jersey, she and Tricia Ann had a messy falling out. Carolyn accused her older sister of trying to steal her son. "You're trying to take my child away from me," she yelled. "You're trying to turn him against me, his mother." The accusations flew heavy and personal. Carolyn was still the baby sister who never quite grew up, who felt as if the world owed her a favor. "You're supposed to be my sister, to love me, no matter what."

After all the years of irresponsibility, how could Tricia Ann truly respond to those accusations coming from the mouth of a drug addict, one relapse away from a crack house? "It was really hard. If she got up there and got settled and was doing well, I would allow him to come for the summer," Tricia Ann recalled.

But her nephew was struggling academically. Tricia Ann tried to explain to Carolyn that, in order to help her son, she needed to get settled first. Tricia Ann was convinced that was the best course of action for Tre, even though it hurt him and his mother even more. "That was difficult for me, knowing he wanted to go with her," she says.

Carolyn moved in with her brother William and got a job at a nursing home. She did well for a few months. Eventually, the boy joined her. Then she called home to Clover, crying. She was upset that her son, the one for whom she wanted to be the best mother, wanted to come home to Tricia Ann and Clover. She also was living without medication. Her noncompliance meant that Carolyn robbed herself of the benefit of all those protease inhibitors on the market that would effectively control the virus and extend her life.

When she returned from New Jersey, she visited the Christopher Clinic and went back on medication. But by then, her fate was sealed. They didn't work for her. Her viral load compared to her T cell counts resembled the score between an NBA team and a third-division college squad. Carolyn gave one last-ditch effort, but it was too late for her.

"She did try," her sister says. Tricia Ann remembers the first time the doctor and social worker told Carolyn that the meds weren't working for her. There was the usual screaming, crying, and hysterics. Then she promptly hit the streets to start abusing drugs again. Sometimes it sounded as if everything that happened in Carolyn's life was an excuse to abuse drugs.

"You don't know how it feels for people to look at you funny and whisper about you," Carolyn said. The drugs took her mind off things, she said. And so did sex. Through her long night's journey with AIDS, Carolyn never denied herself the social comforts of love and lust. She never stopped dating; she was a hustler of the heart. Everybody in Clover knew. The guy she lived with near the end knew. He really liked Carolyn—she was smart and funny.

Of course, Tricia Ann had her doubts. She knew it wasn't going to work for Carolyn and her boyfriend. While he was away at work, Carolyn scoured the neighborhood for drugs. Some nights Tricia Ann encountered her sister walking the streets. On her way to Walmart one night, Tricia Ann saw her sister on the street and inquired about her nephew. Carolyn had left her son in the care of her live-in boyfriend. This was a familiar pattern. At first, it was convenient for her. Then the arguments started. Carolyn spent the rent money on drugs. When her boyfriend began to fuss, it was time for her to move on. Soon afterward the relationship ended.

Despite her criminal past and her drug habits, Carolyn got a welfare check to help support her and her son. But she owed every drug dealer in the neighborhood. On the first of the month, when she received her money, the drug dealers appeared to collect their debts. One weekend in March 2002, one of those drug dealers sold Carolyn a special dose. Her son found his mother in their apartment frothing at the mouth, unconscious. Instinctively, he knew what to do. He took off running for Aunt Tricia Ann's house. She awakened that Sunday morning to the sound of her nephew's frantic cries coming down the path.

"I can't get Momma off the floor," he yelled. "She won't get up." Tricia Ann hurriedly wrapped a robe around herself and followed her nephew back to the apartment. Carolyn lay on the floor, her eyes rolled back into her head. She wore the same clothes she'd had on the night before.

That morning, Tricia Ann and Larry drove behind the ambulance as it raced to Rock Hill. Nothing equals the uncertainty of following an ambulance that is carrying a relative or a spouse. That two-hundred-foot distance is a cruel gap. No doubt Tricia Ann's mind was racing. Would her sister live or die? At Piedmont Medical Center, the emergency room physicians said Carolyn's lifestyle might have caught up with her. Somebody had sold her drugs laced with some unknown, deadly substance.

Since Carolyn was unconscious, she couldn't tell the doctors what drugs she had ingested. Each minute they spent trying to find out was a minute subtracted from Carolyn's life. As she sat in the waiting room, Tricia Ann tried to remember the men Carolyn had been standing with the previous night. One was a known drug dealer. A few days later, Tricia Ann approached him. She was direct.

"Did Carolyn get any drugs from you Saturday night?" she asked. "I know she was up there chillin' with you guys. Just tell me what was in the drugs." The man swore he didn't sell Carolyn any drugs. But his actions betrayed his words. After Carolyn died he offered Tricia Ann some money for Carolyn's son.

At other times, he spoke to the young boy directly and offered him money, but Tricia Ann stopped him. She refused to a let a drug dealer salve his conscience with a few dollars to the son of a woman whose death he might have hastened.

Even as Carolyn lay dying in Rock Hill, about ninety miles to the south, in the South Carolina State House, the fight against AIDS took center stage. State senator John Wesley Matthews Jr., chairman of the South Carolina Legislative Black Caucus, stepped to the podium on the floor of the South Carolina Senate. Matthews, a retired elementary school teacher, sponsored a resolution to honor Dr. Michael Watson, one of his constituents. Resolutions are the dog-and-pony shows of legislative life. Politicians treasure those moments of maximum exposure with minimal political risk. Such events usually generate positive press and earn voter loyalty. Matthews, whose district extended from Orangeburg County south to Bamberg, Hampton,

Colleton, and Dorchester counties, which make up the state's Black Belt, was about to pay homage to an extraordinary man with an equally extraordinary career.

The clerk of the Senate then presented Senate Resolution 1148 honoring Dr. Michael C. Watson, a white physician who had dedicated his entire career to caring for the mostly black, mostly poor people in Bamberg County and had opened the first county health clinic specifically for treating people with AIDS and HIV. Watson, then seventy-six, had just retired and sold the private medical practice he had established as a young doctor fresh out of medical school forty-eight years before.

"To commend and congratulate Dr. Michael C. Watson of Bamberg for his distinguished career as a physician and for his dedication to the medical profession and to extend best wishes to him and his family upon his retirement from the Bamberg County Hospital after more than thirty years of service," the resolution read.

True to his modest outlook, Dr. Watson didn't attend the event.

Carolyn came home from the hospital to die. In her final spring, her rebellion ended. She said she wanted to do the right thing.

"I don't know if the drugs just consumed her, but when she realized what it was doing to her, it was too late. She couldn't turn back the clock," Tricia Ann says.

Carolyn's conversation was littered with talk of regrets. Every day she was alert, she apologized. She constantly begged Tricia Ann for forgiveness. Tricia Ann assured her, "I forgave you a long time ago. I just loved you and wanted you to be well and to be safe. You thought I was trying to keep you down."

Carolyn confessed to stealing her sister's household items to sell for money to buy drugs. But her biggest regrets involved her son: she didn't get to raise him. She thanked Tricia Ann for being a good substitute mother to her nephew. "I know he will be all right. I know you will take care of him and will never let him forget his mom and how much she loved him," she said.

During those last few weeks, a friend from Hickory Grove, a hamlet about fifteen minutes from Clover, came to see Carolyn. By then she had lost her appetite. Food had always mattered to Carolyn, but as her life drained out of her battered body, the thought of some fried chicken and macaroni and cheese no longer put a glint in her eyes. Most days, Tricia Ann tried to encourage her sister to drink the nutritional supplement Ensure. Carolyn's friend was a good cook. Trying to cheer her up, the friend asked Carolyn what she felt like eating. "I want steak and a baked potato," Carolyn said.

So the next day, she brought Carolyn a T-bone steak and a baked potato, but Carolyn struggled to swallow. She chewed the steak slowly and took sips of orange soda to wash down the food. About halfway through, she stopped. She couldn't eat anymore. That was her last bite.

But even with her waning strength, Carolyn tried to assert authority, to be a mother to her son. One day Tremaine came home from school with a poor grade. It didn't matter that Carolyn had never cared about learning, never respected her teachers; she wanted her son to be different. She fussed at him.

"Come here, I'm going to whup you," she said to him. Tricia Ann laughed all the way down into the pit of her stomach at the irony of the exchange between mother and son. She knew her sister didn't have the strength to raise her hand to beat her son. "Hearing her trying to fuss at her son and knowing that her strength was gone, I would look at her and laugh."

Soon afterward, Tricia Ann overheard a conversation between mother and son. Carolyn lay in a hospital bed, while he occupied a twin bed nearby. Carolyn talked to Tre about being a man. "Never be ashamed of who you are," she said. "Never let anyone make you feel ashamed." She stressed the importance of doing well in school. "Get an education and grow up to be a man. Don't let anyone stop you."

The next day Carolyn decided to tape a video to leave for her son. Friends came over with the video equipment, but it was too late. By the time they set up the equipment, Carolyn had slipped into a coma.

During the sisters' last conversation, Carolyn talked about how she wanted the end to be. "I want to die early in the morning with the window cracked to feel the breeze," she said.

"Why?" Tricia Ann asked.

"That's what I want."

On April 30, 2002, Carolyn got her wish.

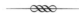

When the doctors sent Carolyn home to die just after Easter, it gave Tricia Ann Starr a new perspective on what it meant to live with a relative dying of AIDS. She had seen others die of the disease, but none of them was her sister. "I wasn't there every day for the others. I wasn't there seven days a week," she told me. With Carolyn, she saw everything, the pain she was in. She saw her baby sister grasping for life. It was just heartbreaking.

Having watched as AIDS slowly killed her sister, Tricia Ann vowed to speak out about the danger of AIDS even more. "I have to, now more so than ever," she said. But as she spoke a few days after Carolyn's death, Tricia Ann as yet didn't understand the power of shame, the culture of silence; it silenced even her at her sister's funeral.

Tricia Ann didn't speak during her sister's funeral service, although she wanted to. She felt young people needed to hear Carolyn's unvarnished truth. Everyone there knew Carolyn had died of AIDS, but no one said it. "Carolyn didn't die a pretty death. She died full of pain," Starr said. "She didn't die of sickle cell, she didn't die of cancer. She died of AIDS."

Even as she buried her baby sister, Tricia Ann did not know that the cycle of pain, anger, and helplessness would soon be repeated again as AIDS stole another member of her family.

22

TRACY

When Dr. Charles sent Carolyn home because there was nothing else he could do for her, Tracy Walker, her niece, stayed with Carolyn at the house every day. Tracy would sit in the room watching her aunt. The day Carolyn died, Tracy climbed into the hospital-issued bed and curled up in a fetal position.

"Aunt Trish, I will be next," she said. "This is where I want to die."

That pronouncement shook Tricia Ann to the depths of her heart. Tracy was Tricia Ann's favorite niece, the daughter of John, Tricia Ann's oldest brother. Tracy was the family's go-to girl. She was the one niece everyone loved. She could be trusted to run an errand. She was the one who made the long trip of more than five hours to eastern North Carolina to get Carolyn the day she was released from a North Carolina prison in 1997 so Carolyn wouldn't have to catch the bus home. If there were bills to pay, family members could trust Tracy to pay them on time and not spend the money on drugs.

But Tracy had been born in 1969. She was just thirty-two. She was still in the prime of her life, and here she was talking about dying. Tricia Ann tried to put a stop to that kind of talk right away.

"I knew I had to get the hospital bed out of my house," Tricia Ann says. She picked up the phone and called the hospital equipment rental company. "They told us they would get the bed the next day. I told them they had to come get the bed the same day."

Tracy had lost hope. She took a blanket and curled up on the floor. A week before the funeral, Tricia Ann had to get firm with Tracy. She had to go home. Tracy accompanied Tricia Ann and Larry to select a casket and a burial site for Carolyn. She was buried not in the black community cemetery but at the family plot outside town. Tracy, the high school graduate, helped write Carolyn's obituary and was assigned the task of notifying Carolyn's old druggie friends that she had died.

The day Tracy walked into Generation Funeral Home to view Carolyn's body, she collapsed to the floor. "I want my aunt Carolyn, I want my aunt Carolyn," she wailed as her father carried her out to the car.

A few days later, at Carolyn's funeral, mourners gathered early. Seats in the sanctuary filled quickly. I attended the funeral accompanied by my wife and two children. I parked my silver Chrysler Concorde in the dirt lot near the rear of the white church and walked up to the building. On my way there, I saw Tracy for the first time in more than a year. I remembered her as a smallish, good-looking, dark-skinned woman who wore her hair pulled tightly back in a neat bun. But the Tracy I saw looked completely different. Her body was bloated, her stomach protruding as if she were six months pregnant.

As I walked into the sanctuary I met Reverend Starr, who was dressed in her Sunday best as she tried to stay dignified to bid farewell to her sister. The words leapt off my tongue. "How come you didn't tell me Tracy was pregnant?" I whispered to Tricia Ann, who responded with a quizzical look.

"Pregnant! Tracy isn't pregnant! It's the AIDS."

Inside, mourners filled every pew and even spilled over into the choir and the dais behind the speakers. Women fanned themselves. As the mourners sat, Tracy stood and walked over to the open casket where Carolyn lay. She wept loud and long, a soulful, heart-searing cry of anguish.

To those who knew her, Tracy was mourning her beloved aunt Carolyn. But to those familiar with her condition, Tracy mourned not for the life just lost but for the road that lay ahead. She looked into the casket and saw her immediate future. She knelt beside the casket, her arms serving as a pillow for her head. Midway through the service, as the men from Generation

Funeral Home stepped forward to close the casket, Tracy tried to get one last glimpse of her aunt. Then, as soon as the lid was closed, she screamed louder and longer, her voice trailing against the backdrop of the songs of praise. After they closed the casket she lay on it and wept.

I had first met Tracy eighteen months before. As fate would have it, on Sunday, December 3, 2000, her face graced the front page of the *Rock Hill Herald*. In the picture Reverend Patricia Ann Starr was talking to L. Z. Witherspoon, a young man from the neighborhood. In the background stood Tracy. She wore no makeup. Her lips were unpainted. Her face was pockmarked with acne. That day, she was playful, smiling and doting on her aunt. She was slim and healthy looking. The photograph had been taken a few days earlier on a Friday afternoon as they stood outside in front of Tricia Ann's house. The photograph was for a story about AIDS in their small town of Clover. Tricia Ann was the focus of the picture and the story. Tracy was supposed to be a prop, just another face in the group, unconnected to the big picture. What I didn't know then was that Tracy was an untold part of the story. She had been diagnosed with the virus years before. Her days were numbered.

Tracy Walker was born mid-November 1969, at the time of year when the leaves had already turned deep orange and when the air in Cloverdale is spiced with the aroma of burning oak firewood. She was the second-to-last child of John, Annie Mae Pegram's oldest son. With four sons and no daughter of her own, Tricia Ann treated Tracy like her daughter. "Coming up, Tracy, she was ours, our little girl."

But at heart, Tracy was a daddy's girl; she loved her father, and he adored her. After her parents broke up, she clung to her father. She also cleaved to her father's side of the family. John didn't say a lot, but he worked hard. Every day when he returned home from work, his boots and pants and shirts showed the signs of a man who had immersed himself wholly in whatever endeavor he chose to make a living that day.

Early on, everyone knew that Tracy, unlike many of her neighbors, would graduate from high school. Then she fell in love with one of her schoolmates. Teen love turned to unprotected sex, a habit that would cost her dearly later on. She became pregnant.

Nothing disrupts a young girl's life like a missed menstrual period and an unplanned, unwanted pregnancy. One day the teenager walked into the Starr house. She was clearly upset—she was crying. She had just had an abortion. In some ways she was still Tracy, but to those who really knew her she was never quite the same again.

After Tracy graduated from Clover High, she found work in Gastonia at Roush's, a manufacturer and distributor of Christmas decorations, then with Bali, a manufacturer of women's underwear in Kings Mountain. While her work life was steady, her social life unraveled. After the abortion, Tracy shared her heart and her body freely. She didn't worry about getting pregnant again because the abortion killed more than her unborn fetus. Something went wrong in that doctor's office. She would never bear children.

Tracy longed for children of her own, but in the absence of that she claimed all her cousins and nieces and nephews as her own. Tracy loved all children, especially Carolyn's son, Tre. He was her heart. When Carolyn went to prison, Tracy took special interest in the jail-orphaned boy. She took him to the movies and skating. Tricia Ann would drop him off, and Tracy would be right there.

Tracy had a persistent girlishness; she never quite grew up. But she was a good role model, too. Tracy wouldn't take the children anywhere unless they were doing well in school. She didn't care for children who were hard-headed or rude or who showed off. During the summer, she loaded the neighborhood children into Uncle Zeb's van and drove them to Vacation Bible School. "Kids really were drawn to Tracy," Tricia Ann says. "It pained her even more not having any of her own."

But just as she loved the children in her extended family, Tracy was also protective of her adult relatives. When her uncle Woody fell ill, Tracy was the faithful, uncomplaining errand girl. "We always depended on Tracy," Tricia Ann says.

But there was a tough side to her generous heart. She didn't shy away from violence. Once a man up the block jumped her brother and beat him up. Her brother was a short, little guy. When Tracy found out, she went after her brother's attacker and stabbed him with a knife. Afterward, Larry called her "Bloody Tracy." "Tracy will cut you, now," he teased. "Don't mess with her."

Tracy was tragically drawn to the wrong guys, like the boyfriend who lent her a coat with a marijuana joint in the pocket. As she drove home from the club on that cold night, she encountered a police roadblock. They stopped her, searched her, and found the stub. They arrested her but dropped the charges after the boyfriend admitted that the marijuana was his. Their relationship fizzled soon afterward.

Then there was the New Yorker she met at the post office. She might have been safer if his face had been plastered on a wanted poster, because he was a city slicker who smelled like trouble from the start. He was always visiting the hospital emergency room. He blamed the flu. Friends and relatives tried to warn Tracy. Something is wrong with this guy, they cautioned. Her heart said otherwise. She loved him. "He's anemic," she said defensively.

"It was always something. He would tell her he had sickle cell. It didn't click. The next thing, he left town. His family came and took him back to New York." As soon as her boyfriend disappeared, the rumors started. Some heard he was in prison for armed robbery. He used to call Tracy collect, but she refused to talk to him. When he was released from prison, he called Tracy and promised to be back in six months. She never saw him. Next thing she heard, he had died of walking pneumonia.

Despite her run of bad luck, Tracy never gave up on love. She started dating a guy named Buster, and before long the couple made wedding plans. But after they were married their union was combustible and quickly turned violent. After he pulled out a gun and threatened to kill her, Tracy ran to her aunt for help. When the two returned to the estranged couple's Gastonia apartment to collect Tracy's clothes, he pointed the gun at Tracy. "Aunt Trish, he's going to shoot me," she screamed.

Tricia Ann stepped in front of her niece and tried to show an air of calm. Inside she prayed hard. "You are not going to shoot," she told Tracy's husband. In her mind, she was "pleading the blood of Jesus."

On the outside, she tried to calm the man. But he seemed maniacal— he said if he couldn't have Tracy, then no one would. While Tricia Ann kept him at bay, she coaxed Tracy to run to safety. Then Tricia Ann heard the sirens. During the commotion, someone had called the police. Tracy's husband heard the sirens too and took off running. By the time the squad cars pulled up, he had disappeared. Tricia Ann asked the police to wait around until Tracy finished packing. The women still felt unsafe. They requested a police escort out of the neighborhood to the South Carolina state line.

That episode ended well. Prayers were answered. But at the time, Tricia Ann had no idea just how many prayers Tracy was going to need. Soon afterward, Tracy started getting sickly. She came down with what looked like the flu and just couldn't seem to shake it. Nothing seemed to work. Then she made an appointment to see an infectious disease specialist. Tricia Ann was cleaning a house in Charlotte when her cell phone rang. A nurse called. Did she know a young woman named Tracy Walker? she asked.

In the background, Tricia Ann could hear Tracy screaming and hollering. It sounded like a person who had just seen their house on fire.

"What's wrong? Tell me what's wrong."

The nurse refused to say. "Please, come right away." Tricia Ann didn't hesitate. She dropped the cleaning cloth and drove straight to Gastonia, where she found Tracy seated in the doctor's office. She was still crying hysterically.

"You have to tell me what's wrong."

Then the doctor walked in. "She's HIV positive," he said. Even before the words died on the doctor's lips, Tricia Ann reached out and just grabbed her niece and held her.

"Leave me with her for a while."

A nurse came in and gave Tracy a sedative, while Tricia Ann just sat there and held her niece's hand. "I love you," she repeated over and over again. But all Tracy seemed to remember were the words "HIV positive."

"I'm going to die. People are going to talk about me," she whimpered. She didn't want to tell anyone.

"Tracy, your mommy and daddy need to know," Tricia Ann said. Instead, Tracy made her aunt promise not to say anything until she was ready. But Tricia Ann had walked this road before. She was more concerned about the physical consequences of Tracy's HIV diagnosis than the local gossip in Cloverdale.

"You need to get help," she said. "Let me take you to the clinic." A few days later, Tricia Ann drove Tracy to the Christopher Clinic half an hour away in Rock Hill, where they met with Linda Ashley and Dr. Lackey. That distance was inconvenient, but it made things easier if Tracy wanted to keep her illness a secret.

"Linda couldn't visit her at the house," Tricia Ann says.

Tracy and her aunt kept their secret for a whole year. It was hard, because Tricia Ann had always been close to John, Tracy's father. They talked daily. They confided in each other. Many times, as they sat together and talked, Tricia Ann barely managed to stop herself from divulging Tracy's secret. But it was a special favor for a special niece. Finally, Tricia Ann told her niece that she had to tell her parents. They couldn't keep the truth secret any longer. But Tracy refused. She wanted Tricia Ann to tell them.

So on the weekend Tricia Ann broke the news to John and Peggy, Tracy left town. She couldn't bear to see her parents' reaction when they heard that their daughter had HIV and would likely die of AIDS. So many of their neighbors had endured the physical and social torture inflicted by AIDS. Carolyn had taken that hard road. So had Cliff, Sandy, Jackie, and Nita. Now it would be their dear daughter's turn.

Tracy's mother and father knew that she had been sickly, but neither parent would have ever suspected the extent of their daughter's illness. As preparation for the meeting, Tricia Ann asked John to meet her at his ex-wife's house. Although the couple had been divorced for years, they were still cordial to each other. When Tricia Ann arrived, she almost panicked. Tracy's older sister was in the house. That wasn't part of the plan.

"I'm here to talk to your momma and daddy," she told her.

The young woman didn't back down. "Whatever you tell them you can tell me too," she said insolently. "Anyways, my momma's going to tell me."

Tricia Ann had rehearsed the words in her mind. She told them Tracy needed them more than she ever had in her life. Tracy had AIDS.

"How long?" John asked. He was a man of few words.

"For a year. Tracy didn't want anyone to know. She felt as if you would treat her different," Tricia Ann told them. "She's ashamed, and she needs her family's support."

Tracy returned home that Monday. She knew they would have questions. But she didn't want to talk about it. She didn't want to answer their questions.

Tracy proved to be a frustrating case for Linda Ashley. She didn't like taking the medicine, even though the pills didn't carry the same old side effects. Linda thought Tracy would be a poster girl for HIV and AIDS. She could reach young people.

But Tracy would never be the poster child for AIDS in Clover. She wanted to hide in shame. She hid in the open. As her shame mounted, despair overwhelmed her. Twice she tried to commit suicide. The first time, she ran her car off Highway 55 on the way toward Kings Mountain. The vehicle left the two-lane highway and ran through the woods and into a tree. Tracy was knocked unconscious but escaped any significant injuries.

After that, her parents committed her to get mental health treatment at Gaston Memorial. She did OK for a while, then came home. Depression set in. When lesions appeared on Tracy's face, her neighbors began to speculate about her condition. She couldn't handle it. Her depression worsened. She tried to commit suicide again by overdosing on pills. Her father found her unconscious with the bottle lying beside her and called 911.

Even as Tracy battled depression, she often sought refuge at Tricia Ann's home, where Carolyn lived at the time. Carolyn was walking the final mile of her AIDS journey, and Tracy would sit at the foot of her bed and talk. Carolyn lay in the hospital bed while Tracy was on the twin bed. Sometimes Tracy stayed over, and Tricia Ann would hear Tracy and Carolyn talking late into the night. There is no transcript of those conversations, but one can only imagine their words were peppered with regret, shame, and hurt.

As her condition worsened, Tracy cut off contact with her friends and former coworkers. Her folks might have encouraged the isolation. They didn't want people to visit Tracy, then return to the street to gossip about her. They even discouraged friends from visiting. One visitor who Tracy never refused was Girard Lindsay, a young, dreadlocked bank executive who lived up the street. Girard drove a red Ford Mustang. He had been HIV positive since 1997. Girard took his meds, and he tried in vain to convince Tracy to take hers too. He wanted her to fight for her life, but she didn't want to.

Tracy's isolation meant some members of the Pegram clan didn't know about her condition. Near the end, her uncles and aunts and close friends were devastated when they learned belatedly that Tracy was deathly ill. They were hurt that she hadn't had enough faith in them to tell them. They believed they could have helped her get through this. Tricia Ann couldn't tell them, even if she had wanted to.

"Tracy tied my hands. I had signed a commitment," she says. "I couldn't tell anyone without her permission. She was very selective in who she wanted to know."

Near the end, dementia stole Tracy's memories. She lost her desire to speak. Only the sound of children's voices elicited any joy in her eyes. On trips to the Christopher Clinic, Tricia Ann or John placed her in the wheelchair and wheeled her in. In the fall of 2002, when she was again admitted to Piedmont Medical Center, Tracy was tired of the smell of medicines, of the food, of being sick—period. She told Dr. Charles just how she felt.

"I'm not coming back," she said. That was the same day her family's pastor came to visit. As he walked in, Tracy's eyes were closed as if she were either asleep or unconscious, but she wasn't. "Do you know who I am?" he asked. "I am your pastor."

Even as she was dying, she could never suffer fools gladly. "You're not my pastor," Tracy replied. "You're my momma's pastor. That's my pastor over there," she said, pointing to Tricia Ann, who was seated near the bed.

After she was discharged that final time, whenever Tracy needed medical care, instead of heading for the hospital, her aunt or her father drove her to the Christopher Clinic. Inside, they wheeled her down to the end of the hallway, turned in to an examination room, and hoisted her thin frame onto the table to wait for Dr. Charles.

Their last visit didn't go well. Dr. Charles walked in to see the patient, but he couldn't get Tracy's blood pressure. Tricia Ann remembered looking at the physician. He had that expression, the same one he wore when he had walked into Carolyn's hospital room eight months earlier. When Tricia Ann saw that look, she could feel the dam of emotions about to give way.

"Excuse me for a minute," she said, as she stepped out of the room and walked down the hallway, away from the exam room, away from the news she was trying to avoid. When her legs could take her no farther, she slumped down on the floor of the hallway and wept. "Not again, God. Not again," she sobbed. "It's too soon."

Sensing a moment of crisis, Dr. Charles stepped out of the examination room, followed Tricia down the hallway, and sat on the floor next to her. He put his arms around her. "We're going to get through this," he said.

"I can't go through this again," she wept.

"It's going to be all right," he tried to reassure her. Dr. Charles knew the next step and broached it carefully. He offered to call hospice for Tracy; there was nothing else he could do for her. Tricia Ann understood immediately that Tracy had made her irreversible downward turn. Tricia Ann had walked that journey with Carolyn. Now she would do so again for her niece. But how would Tracy's father handle it?

"John is not going to go for this. Not hospice," she thought. Months earlier, when Tricia Ann had summoned hospice to care for Carolyn, John was pretty upset. Carolyn had shown signs of a rebound after she was released from the hospital and sent home to die. For him, hospice meant giving up, that there was no hope.

"When we brought in hospice for Carolyn, he had a fit," Tricia Ann recalled. But before hospice, she had to take Tracy home and break the news to her father. "It was what was best for her," she says. "It was hard to keep trying to take her back and forth to the clinic."

Within a day or so, the hospice nurses arrived at Tracy's mother's house. They were the same nurses who had cared for Carolyn the previous spring. Tracy remembered them. She wouldn't talk to them. She wouldn't talk to anyone. Her lips seemed sealed shut by impending doom.

Then amid all the silence, one of Tracy's baby nephews came in.

"Hey, Boo, come to Aunt Tracy." She spoke loud enough for the whole house to hear. She loved children until the end.

That Saturday, Larry visited Tracy. The two always enjoyed sparring with each other. "I didn't get to ride in the big truck, Uncle Larry," Tracy told him. At the time, Larry drove long-haul cargo in his tractor-trailer.

"When I come back, I'll lift you up and put you in the truck," he promised. But time stole his chance to fulfill that pledge.

With her days dwindling, Tracy finally allowed her mother, Peggy, to baby her and love her in a way she never had before. Tricia Ann was tired; she had stayed up with Tracy for days. She went home and was about to go to bed.

Peggy called. She was crying. "I can't stay here without you."

So Tricia Ann returned and slept on the floor. Around 4:00 AM on November 2, 2002, she awoke to hear Tracy's breathing grow heavy, then subside into an easy, slow, deliberate rhythm. Tricia Ann realized that Tracy had made her final lap.

"It won't be long now," Tricia Ann thought to herself. That realization pushed away sleep, and she rose to wake up Tracy's mother. She then walked down the street to fetch Tracy's father. Then they summoned Tracy's siblings—a brother lived in Morganton, North Carolina, more than sixty miles away. They told him to come by seven o'clock.

When her brother arrived, Tracy heard his voice and opened her eyes. Tricia Ann asked the others to give the two some time alone. Tracy and her brother were always close. A few minutes later, Tricia Ann heard crying inside the bedroom. Tracy's brother was an emotional wreck. They urged him to keep his composure for Tracy's sake.

When calm returned to the house, Tricia Ann washed and changed Tracy. As she did, Tracy began to shake like one of those women in the choir on Sunday at the Fire Baptized Holiness Church.

"Baby, what's wrong?" her mother asked.

Tricia Ann knew. "It was the Holy Ghost. She began to speak in tongues like I've never heard." Tricia Ann looked on in amazement, but Tracy's mother was perturbed. Worshipers didn't behave like that on Sundays at their United Methodist Church.

"What's happening to my baby?" Tracy's mother asked again.

"She is talking to the Father and going home," Tricia Ann replied. Tracy spoke in tongues for ten minutes, like a worshiper at a southern summer tent revival. Then she was silent. She stopped breathing. She sighed, and then she was gone.

"It was a beautiful sight," Tricia Ann says. "This was the Holy Spirit. Tracy always wanted to be baptized with the Holy Ghost."

Six months and two days after Carolyn died, God granted Tracy's wish. Now each November as thoughts turn toward Thanksgiving, Tracy's father and relatives gather in her memory and hold a pig pickin' party. Tracy was thirty-three.

23

A CALL TO ACTION

Tracy Walker's death on November 2, 2002, served as another frustrating reminder to Linda Ashley and the York County AIDS advocacy community of the task ahead. Despite the gains made in the treatment of the disease, too many men and women were still dying of AIDS in small southern towns. And outside the region, few people seemed to notice or care. During the two decades since the arrival of AIDS, the plight of poor, rural men and women with AIDS and HIV always seemed less important, less of a priority, than the suffering in large cities and even in sub-Saharan Africa.

But there were radical plans to change that.

Less than two weeks after Tracy's funeral in Clover, AIDS/STD directors from the states of the Old Confederacy convened forty minutes away in Charlotte for the Southern AIDS Summit. Seated at the table along with the Southern States AIDS/STD Directors Work Group were representatives from the national AIDS director's organization and the Kaiser Family Foundation, a California-based philanthropic organization that dealt with health care policy.

The two-day gathering attracted state health directors, legislators, community activists, and people with AIDS from the Carolinas, Mississippi, Alabama, Texas, Louisiana, Florida, Virginia, and Washington, DC, to review the AIDS crisis in the South.

Those who had led the perennial struggle against sexually transmitted diseases in the South had tackled HIV and AIDS head-on. For twenty years they had toiled largely in obscurity, while activists from the big cities grabbed the limelight, headlines, and funding. Finally, they were fed up with the status quo and fed up with their national organization. A year earlier, unhappy with the national group, they had formed their own regional group to raise an alarm about the growing epidemic in the South.

At the Charlotte event, the former surgeon general Dr. David Satcher delivered the keynote address to members, who during those few days decided that the southern states should focus their efforts on lobbying Washington for more money "because of the unfair funding distribution." The gathering also served as a warm-up for the Southern AIDS Conference, which attracted more than one hundred community activists, care agency leaders, and government health employees in Tampa, Florida, two weeks later.

A key element of the strategy was to generate media coverage of the issue. And the lynchpin of that strategy was the *Southern States Manifesto*. That weekend in Tampa, the group endorsed the manifesto and created the Southern AIDS Coalition, which would become the South's vanguard in the uncivil war between the nation's regions over the allocation of scarce federal Ryan White CARE Act funds four years later.

"We all basically said, 'We've got to do something,'" said Kathie Hiers, director of AIDS Alabama, a private nonprofit based in Birmingham. Hiers, along with Evelyn Foust of the North Carolina Department of Health and Human Services, cochaired the Southern AIDS Coalition for about five years. "The Tampa meeting got us fired up," she recalls. "After that first manifesto, we got serious and really geared up the group."

It required months of revisions, but the *Southern States Manifesto* was finally released on March 2, 2003. On the cover is a map of the southern half of the United States, from DC in the northeast to Texas in the southwest. The forty-two-page document sought to highlight a long-festering sore on the national health care landscape.

Although AIDS began in the large cities of New York and California in 1981, twenty-two years later the disease, like a slow-moving demographic algae bloom, had fanned across America's rural hamlets and towns. The color and gender of the illness had changed. People like Linda Ashley and

Patricia Ann Starr knew it years before. Finally, the region demanded that the rest of the country acknowledge it.

"Over the last decade, the HIV/AIDS and STD epidemics continue to increase in every southern locality, particularly among poor, disenfranchised, and minority populations. Southern state governments and localities are struggling to find resources for disease prevention and care and treatment for the growing number of people living with HIV/AIDS and/or STDs," Southern State AIDS Directors Work Group cochairs, Evelyn Foust and Beth Scalco, stated in the manifesto. "It is urgent that federal, state, and local governments and leaders in local communities recognize the disparate impact of HIV and STDs in the South."

This "Call to Action," like the cannon ball hurled at Fort Sumter 140 years before, was just the first volley of what would soon become a three-year war, not just between states but between the regions, south and northeast, urban and rural, over the equitable allocation of money to pay for the sick and dying afflicted with HIV and AIDS.

"The Deep South is driving the epidemic. Our mortality outcomes are still extremely high," Hiers says. "All the other regions of the country have gone down in double digits; ours have not. It's very frustrating."

Linda Ashley worked hard. For five years she had slaved as the director of the Christopher Clinic, one of the first privately run, nonprofit, full-service HIV and AIDS care providers in the state. Agency heads from all over the Southeast called to ask how to replicate the clinic's success. The clinic paid very little rent thanks to the generosity of the landlord. With the help of a five-year, $2 million Ryan White CARE Act grant, the agency quadrupled its staff to sixteen employees on the payroll. With the grant money the clinic also secured Dr. Charles's services as medical director and covered the cost of medication and other services for hundreds of men and women living with AIDS.

All was going well. Or so Linda thought when she boarded a flight with her friend Mickey for a three-week vacation in Alaska. America's north country still had enough of summer for the vacationers to enjoy long days and nights. Those idyllic three weeks with all of Alaska's lakes and teeming wildlife must have reminded Linda of her wonderful childhood in Jacksonville, Florida. She returned home from her vacation with a suitcase filled with gifts for her loyal staff.

Upon her return home, one item of business for her first week back was a meeting with the board of directors. She had personally invited each of the members to serve. Before the meeting, Linda ran her numbers and prepared the financial reports. She had recently let the agency's accountant go. As she headed for the boardroom, money was not one of her worries. Her thoughts must have been about what vacation highlights she should share with her board members. After all, this was just another routine board meeting, like the many she had attended over the previous five years. Several of the board members were out of town and would be absent for the 5:30 PM weekday meeting, but that was not unusual given the time of year.

As Linda walked into the meeting room, nothing seemed amiss, but she should have noticed that, after not seeing her for three weeks, the board members were less than effusive in their greetings. Some even looked away, seemingly uncomfortable to meet her gaze. In the South, small talk usually precedes business. But that August afternoon, none of the usual pleasantries were exchanged. The room took on a subtle quiet.

There are moments in life when you can look back and recall obvious clues to oncoming danger. That was one of those moments for Linda. But the survival instincts that had kept her alive through an abusive marriage and saved her after her son's suicide must have been dulled from the success of the previous five years. She should have noticed that none of the board members looked at her. They averted their eyes as if to avoid being distracted from what they were about to do next. As she sat at the head of the table, board chairman Michael Laessle announced a special agenda item the directors needed to discuss.

Laessle had joined the Catawba Care Coalition board the previous year and made a splash with a $250,000 donation to the agency. Records show that in March 2000, he created the Michael D. Laessle AIDS Foundation.

As board chairman, Laessle was closely involved in overseeing the agency. He came by regularly. He endearingly called Linda his "Earth Angel."

That day, however, Laessle had no terms of endearment for his executive director. He announced that while Linda was on vacation a consultant conducted a survey of the Christopher Clinic employees. Some of the longtime staff members didn't quite understand the point of the questions, but the consultant had done what the chairman called a "weather report" of the agency.

For Linda, the forecast was seismic. The employees were unhappy with the way she ran the clinic, the chairman said. "It's time for you to go," someone, perhaps the chairman, said to Linda. She could either resign or be fired.

"I was totally caught off guard," she says. Laessle slid a letter in front of her to sign. Details of all that was said are scant. She felt defenseless. Her strongest supporters on the board were absent. No one at the table spoke up for her. "It was a coup."

Laessle demanded Linda's keys to the building. The board forbade her to contact any of the clinic's employees or risk her severance. The chairman walked her to the door. She could return on Saturday to collect her personal things from the office when no other employees were present. "By the time I got to my car, I was just sobbing," Linda says.

When the employees showed up for work the next morning, board members were there to greet them. "Linda will not be back," was all the board members told the clinic employees.

A few days later, when the absent board members returned, they were displeased with her firing, but they were outnumbered. There was little they could do. "It was a done deal," Linda says.

That Saturday, Linda drove to the Camden Avenue office to retrieve her things. A board member let her into her office and stood watch while Linda packed her art and personal items, as if she would steal or damage the clinic she had worked so hard to build.

After she collected her possessions in a box, she carried out her rocking chair and handmade blanket. Those were her two comfort tools the lecturers in graduate school had never told her about. When men and women came into her office to talk about their battle with AIDS, Linda would let them sit in the rocker and wrap the blanket around themselves. Now she herself needed the solace of her rocker and purple afghan, but for months she would not find it.

In South Carolina, a right-to-work state, labor laws are stacked overwhelmingly in favor of employers. After all, this was a state that was always dominated by the landed and moneyed class. Still, Linda figured she had rights. How could a bunch of volunteers, whom she had handpicked, fire her without warning, without anything more solid than an unscientific survey of employees?

Wasn't she the one who had filed the nonprofit incorporation papers and secured tax-exempt status?

Wasn't she the person who had found the location for the clinic and convinced the landlord to go easy on the rent?

She had found the infectious disease doctor and filled out the reams of paperwork to apply for the Ryan White CARE Act grant, which brought $400,000 a year into the agency's coffers.

Linda consulted an attorney who told her it was useless. "This happens," he said. For weeks she was ashamed to leave her house. Rock Hill is a small place. After all, in a small southern town rumors flew. Everyone knew Linda was the "AIDS lady." People would speculate. They would think she was fired because she stole money. "Word was going around town like wildfire," she says.

Linda also fretted about the suitcase filled with gifts she had brought back from Alaska. "I couldn't even give them out after the trip. It was crazy," she says. "I was upset for myself, but I was upset for the employees. What are they going to think? I can't even talk to them." It felt so unfair in so many ways. "I couldn't face anybody," she laments. "I didn't get to say good-bye to the clients."

In desperation, she visited her pastor, Reverend Bob Shrum, the liberal minister of the progressive-leaning Oakland Baptist Church. The congregation had donated space for a pantry to store supplies for people with HIV and AIDS. Members volunteered to care for people with AIDS. Shrum tried to help Linda put things into perspective. "This kind of thing happens all the time," he told her. "It won't be the last time. It has to do with power."

"I don't get it," she replied.

"What you need to know is that you will be OK," he tried to reassure her. "There will be something better." Those words brought her scant comfort.

She cried for the next few weeks. Finally, she pulled herself together long enough to file for unemployment. The agency's board fought her claim, but she won. But unemployment insurance and a modest severance couldn't salve the bitter betrayal she felt during those first few months after her ouster. "At that point I was totally devastated," she says. "I went into a cave."

Linda didn't have to wait long to find out where her beloved agency was headed. On September 19, Anita Case, whom Linda had hired years earlier, walked in and sat down at Linda's old desk. Case had served as the Christopher Clinic's case management supervisor for three years but had left twelve months earlier to work as an HIV prevention supervisor for Hope Health Inc. in Florence, South Carolina.

In announcing the new director, on October 5, 2005, the *Rock Hill Herald* reported that the Christopher Clinic was positioning itself for the future and was about to launch a capital campaign so the agency would need to rely less on grants to make up its $1.4 million budget. Chairman Laessle said he hoped people would donate money to match his six-figure gift to the agency. "It's a new era," Laessle told the *Herald*. "It's very exciting. We've grown so much."

At that time, 342 persons with AIDS and HIV visited the clinic for treatment. Those numbers represented over 40 percent of the 763 people living with AIDS or HIV in the three-county region served by the Catawba Care Coalition's clinic. "It's a sanctuary, a place where people will love you and care for you," Laessle told the *Herald*. "It's a very nurturing place."

The 520-word *Herald* article touted all the innovations Case had planned for the agency but made no mention of Linda Ashley, either as former or founding director of the clinic. It was as if she had never worked there. Likewise the agency's website makes no mention of Ashley's contributions.

It was as if she had been purged from the agency's institutional memory.

At 3:00 PM on Wednesday, March 1, 2006, in the Dirksen Senate Office Building, Chairman Mike Enzi, a Wyoming Republican, called a Senate Health, Education, Labor, and Pensions Committee (HELP) hearing: "Fighting the AIDS Epidemic of Today: Revitalizing the Ryan White CARE Act."

The legislation had been enacted in 1990 and named for the Indiana hemophiliac teen who had contracted HIV from a tainted blood transfusion three years earlier. It was considered to be a belated but "comprehensive approach to the provision of medical care, treatment and support services to individuals living with HIV/AIDS who have no other means to obtain such care."

Every five years the law came up for renewal. Congress amended and reauthorized the legislation in 1996 and in 2000. At the time of the hearing, the current authorization of appropriation had expired six months earlier, on September 30, 2005. That such a vital and bipartisan piece of legislation remained in limbo half a year after it lapsed was a testament to the contentious and divisive issues that turned former allies into bitter antagonists.

As committee staff prepped Room 430 for the hearing, a line gathered outside the door. On that late winter afternoon in Washington, seats were at a premium. The HELP Committee was scheduled to hear testimony from Bush administration official Dr. Elizabeth Duke, head of the Health Resources and Services Administration, which is part of the US Department of Health and Human Services. She was a high-profile witness, and there were not nearly enough seats to accommodate the large numbers of AIDS industry officials in Washington. At 3:04 PM, Chairman Enzi banged his gavel and opened the hearing.

"If he were alive today, Ryan White would be a witness to the world that has changed a great deal in terms of those affected by HIV and AIDS and the treatment and care. He would celebrate the new, life-saving drugs, which have meant that the safety net program no longer just helps people die with grace and dignity, but it focuses each day on saving lives through treatment," Enzi read. The second-term senator then set the tone of the debate and hinted at the fault lines shaping up in the battle over funding.

"However, to defeat this disease, we have to focus on the epidemic of today and not yesterday." That was an oblique reference to the urban versus rural standoff in the fight to shift additional money to areas outside the large cities. These areas, like small-town Clover, were being forced to respond to the AIDS epidemic without the resources, know-how, or facilities to do so. But if those in the hearing room missed the hint, Enzi, a former shoe store owner, came straight to the point. "Here in the United States, this disease affects more women, more minorities, and more people in rural areas than ever before."

Enzi cited the Kaiser Family Foundation statistics, which showed that more African Americans were affected and dying from HIV than any other ethnic or racial group in the United States. Black folks such as Girard Lindsay and Robbie Hall of Clover represented half of all AIDS diagnoses in 2004, compared with only 25 percent in 1986.

Early in the epidemic, relatively few women were diagnosed with HIV infection and AIDS. But twenty-five years later, the CDC data showed that "the HIV/AIDS epidemic represents a growing and persistent health threat to women in the United States, especially young and minority women. African American women account for two-thirds of the new AIDS cases among women," Enzi said in his opening statement.

"Finally, the epidemic is moving south. Seven of the states with the ten highest AIDS case rates are located in the South," Chairman Enzi said. "Our response must acknowledge these demographic shifts so that we can ensure equitable treatment for all Americans living with HIV.

"Our federal resources for HIV, including those we provide through the Ryan White CARE Act, should go to where the epidemic is today and will be tomorrow—not necessarily where it was a decade ago. If we are to ensure equity, however, we have to first understand the current inequities within the system."

Senator Enzi had thrown down the gauntlet. As a representative from a rural, sparsely populated state, he was putting folks from places like New York, California, New Jersey, and Massachusetts on notice that the landscape had changed. After Enzi finished his statement, Senator Edward Kennedy, the committee's ranking Democrat, then took a turn at the microphone.

"As we increase our efforts to provide better care and treatment and drugs in rural areas that have seen an increase in the AIDS epidemic, we must ensure that more state flexibility does not cause the collapse of existing structures of care under Ryan White," Kennedy warned, his glasses perched low on his nose as he read. "The Ryan White CARE Act is about more than just funds and health care services. It is about caring and the American tradition of reaching out to people who are suffering and in need of help."

Both Enzi and his Democratic colleague stressed the need for a bipartisan, open, collaborative approach on this critical issue. But those familiar with the deal making before and after that hearing said the deliberations were conducted behind closed doors with little input from the people who knew most about the problem. Critics complained that the Republican majority staff locked down the process in a way that restricted access to the groups who advocated for AIDS funding. That had never happened before.

"It wasted time. It was disrespectful. It was counterproductive. At the end it didn't work," recalls Ernest Hopkins of the San Francisco AIDS Foundation. "They had a bad habit of swearing staff to secrecy. They could tell no one."

Senators Enzi and Kennedy agreed to craft legislations as partners. But critics said the cards were stacked in the Republican's favor. "Many of the provisions that we didn't support were provisions that came from Enzi's side," Hopkins said. "His staffers decided to put them in instead of working for a compromise."

Outside the halls of Congress, it got really nasty. Kathie Hiers of AIDS Alabama and other members of the Southern AIDS Coalition arrived early for one committee hearing to stand in line so they could get seats. As the southerners waited to enter the hearing room, representatives from several national AIDS organizations walked up and entered the line ahead of those waiting. "They just broke in front of us in line," Hiers recalled. "They were just rude."

One of the southerners objected. "It's a small room, but I hope we all get in." Those who broke into the line didn't even turn around to acknowledge the aggrieved.

"They were there with lobbyists. We can't afford lobbyists. We have to do the work ourselves," Hiers said. "The national groups were threatened by the Southern AIDS Coalition."

That minor spat typified the rivalry among those who made a living caring and advocating for people with AIDS. Former allies turned on each other in a zero sum game of intraregional backbiting. Old friendships and alliances had become frayed as states and regions lined up to secure their share of AIDS funds. They competed for the same pot of money. If the South won, the Northeast, West, and Midwest lost.

"All of my colleagues from up North said, 'It's not right to shift money from one place to another,'" Hiers recalled. This was no mere polite difference of opinion. "I got a death threat," Hiers says. "I had people following me at conferences calling me liar."

The rhetoric became increasingly shrill as both sides accused each other of playing dirty. "With the same pot of money one jurisdiction had spent Ryan White funding to produce a gold lamé poetry book," Hiers says. "We couldn't get antiretrovirals. They paid for acupuncture and massages, in the past even dog walking and gym memberships."

Conservative Republicans saw it as an opportunity to attack Democrats who represented largely urban areas of the country. Some of the staunchest supporters of AIDS funding, such as Senator Hillary Clinton and House Speaker Nancy Pelosi, voted against the bill, expressing distaste for the altered funding formulas that seem to take money away from places like New York City and San Francisco.

On May 17, the Senate HELP Committee finally introduced and passed the reauthorization bill SR 2823. On September 21, the House of Representatives introduced HR 6143, which passed seven days later by 325 to 98 votes. Representative Gregory Meeks and the entire New York delegation voted against the Ryan White reauthorization.

In a statement released the next day, September 29, 2006, Meeks, a member of the Congressional Black Caucus, predicted New York City would lose more than $17 million from the legislation and that minorities, the poor, and the uninsured "will most seriously suffer."

"New York's health care community and the HIV/AIDS population will face catastrophic losses," he warned.

According to the Congressional Budget Office, the authorization was estimated to cost taxpayers $2.3 billion for fiscal year 2007 and $12.2 billion over the four-year period 2007 to 2011. Even though the program expired in 2005, about $2 billion was allocated to pay for fiscal year 2006, so there would be no break in programs.

The bill included grants to local governments based on the number of people living with HIV and AIDS. It would require agencies that get grants to spend 75 percent of the money on primary care; it provided core medical services grants to states to finance the AIDS Drug Assistance Program, which pays for antiretroviral medicines; it paid for the early diagnostic programs and early intervention systems run by community-based nonprofits such as the Catawba Care Coalition and its Christopher Clinic. Provisions were also added to have funds for women and children with HIV and AIDS.

Supporters of the act argued that with HIV/AIDS no longer localized in the cities as in the early 1980s, rural areas were being punished for being affected later. Southern states had 46 percent of all new AIDS cases but received only 34 percent of funding because they have fewer metropolitan areas that qualified for city grants. They charged that New York people with HIV and AIDS faced no wait for lifesaving drugs and could take advantage of a range of support services not available for people in rural areas, according to the December 2006 *Congressional Digest*.

With House passage of the bill, supporters thought that the Senate would follow suit. But opponents blocked attempts by Enzi to bring the legislation to the Senate floor. New York senators Hillary Clinton and Charles Schumer and New Jersey senators Frank Lautenberg and Robert Menendez placed "holds" on the bill, thus preventing the full Senate from proceeding with debate and vote under a unanimous consent agreement, the December 2006 *Congressional Digest* reported.

The solution, critics argued, was for Congress to allocate more money to meet new demands for treatment and services. "The recent debate around the Ryan White CARE Act has been marred by misconceptions and mired in politics," said Senator Clinton during debate on the floor of the Senate. "There are those making misleading statements about my state—that we misuse funding or do not use the funding we receive, claims that are simply not true."

The strategy being deployed by the bill's supporters was divisive, Clinton argued. "There are those suggesting that somehow the epidemic has changed, trying to pit one part of the country against another, trying once again to divide us," she said. The answer, she said, was more funding. "Let's put our money where our mouth is," she continued. "Let's put money into this program so we are not picking between a poor African American in New York City and a poor African American woman in Alabama."

One major change was that old funding was based on the number of AIDS cases, which gave localities hit hard early by AIDS an advantage in the race for money. The 2006 bill called for the inclusion of both AIDS and HIV cases, which allowed for those areas recently hit by HIV infection to respond more quickly to the coming epidemic.

The Ryan White CARE Act of 2006 marked a major victory for the rural areas and the Southern AIDS Coalition in particular. They had argued successfully that the South bore a larger burden of AIDS and HIV than the funding mechanism paid for.

"They were counting every person with the disease from the beginning, but only those with AIDS, dead or alive. That artificially keeps the money in San Francisco and New York," said Kathie Hiers. "By not counting HIV they are punishing the South."

With both sides deadlocked, the Senate adjourned on September 30, thus missing the October 1 deadline for reauthorization. Negotiations resumed during the lame duck session of Congress after the midterm elections, when Democrats prepared to take control of the Senate and strengthened their hold on the House of Representatives.

Late on the night of December 6, the Senate passed a compromise bill, HR 6143. Kathie Hiers was ensconced in a hotel room in New Orleans watching the vote streaming across her laptop. "I was screaming when it got passed in the wee hours of the morning," she says.

Three days later, the House passed the Senate version of HR 6143 on a voice vote. Christmas came six days early for supporters of the bill when President Bush signed the Ryan White CARE Act Reauthorization into law. Unlike earlier versions, the bill was good for three years instead of five. It sunset in 2009 instead of 2011, the thirtieth anniversary of the outbreak of AIDS.

"It was not a great bill. It was truncated. No one was satisfied," said Hopkins. "Everyone thought it was a flawed product. But it was what it was."

The "Southern victory" was accomplished by an unlikely alliance between Dixie AIDS activists and a cadre of conservative Republican senators: Jeff Sessions from Alabama, Tom Coburn from Oklahoma, Robert Burr from North Carolina, and Chairman Enzi of Wyoming. Conservatives had found common cause with gay and AIDS activists in the unlikely realm of regional solidarity, South against Northeast, rich versus poor, city versus country, and won.

"They said it was not right," Hiers says. "They really fought for us."

24

ROBBIE

Thick leaden clouds hid the sun, banishing its warmth. The gray after-noon was cold and damp. It didn't help that the trees were all shorn of leaves, leaves that fluttered and jumped in the gutters as sedans and dark SUVs drove west on State Road 5 past Black's farm stand and the peach orchards and turned left on Cedar Grove Road past modular houses with paddocks and grazing animals.

As the road meandered southward, stands of oak hugged the side of the highway. A cluster of houses gave way to a clearing, and a white wooden church swung into view. Cars and pickup trucks occupied the grass parking lot, more fallen leaves than grass. Inside, a sad chorus rang out. A blue casket sat in a place of honor in the front between the first row of pews and the pulpit. Mourners dressed in gray wool suits and black leather jackets huddled tightly inside the small space. Others walked inside and stood over the open casket.

Robbie Hall lay in repose, dressed in a black pinstripe suit and white shirt. His head was bald in life and in death. His features were thin and shrunken, the face of a seventy-year-old man. But Robbie's life was cut short at forty-nine. That day the church's furnace refused to light. There was no heat inside the sanctuary except the warmth generated by the flames from two portable kerosene heaters placed on either side toward the front of the church. In the kerosene heater on the right, reddish orange flames flickered and jumped in a vain attempt to dispel the cold seeping inside.

The raised platform was split in three. On the left sat choir members dressed in black, their lapels adorned with festive red ribbons, a symbol of solidarity in the fight against AIDS. In the middle, two women, one wearing glasses and the long, black gown of clergy, sat next to two men dressed in black suits. To the right, another group, one man and several women, sat like a second choir. In the front row, Bobby Johnson, his hair gray with age, kept the song alive. Each time the chorus died, his deep, guttural voice rose again; his right foot stomped in time; the floorboards shook and groaned to life in a liturgical call and response for the ages.

Voices of Deliverance, six Charleston singers accompanied by pianist Howard Brown, sang. The choral group filled the room as if they were a mass choir of a hundred voices.

Leaning on the everlasting arms.

Floorboards shook. Leather shoes stomped.

The Lord is my shepherd.

The congregation of mourners broke into song again.

You are my refuge.

When I call you answer.

As if by rote the mourners rose en masse, their feet stomped in time; the floorboards shook again and recoiled. In one pew, all the men wore dark shades. On a cloudy day, sunglasses aren't to protect the eyes. They hide tears along with the fear and anxiety that attends another funeral for a friend, maybe a former lover, felled by AIDS.

I will not fear the terror by night for angels are encamped around me, they sang.

"I trust you, Lord," someone shouted.

I will not fear the terror by day.

Carolyn Brown's soprano rose in a crescendo. But there seemed to be a vacuum, a missing voice, an emptiness Robbie's tenor usually filled. Brown first met Robbie in 1983 in the play *Ain't Misbehavin'.* "He was always about singing," she said. "He loves to sing." She spoke of Robbie in the present tense, as if the man whose voice had lifted hers for the past decade would never be stilled, never be silent.

Robbie was a young man blessed with talent, she said. The twenty-third psalm was his favorite Bible verse. But his repertoire was usually secular. He sang with the bands Rivers & Company and Black Velvet. He graced the stage for the Charleston Actors Theater.

Reverend Starr stepped forward to the lectern. She had known Robbie his entire life. Robbie was from Armstrong Street in Cloverdale. Unlike so many young men raised by teenage mothers, Robbie was a good boy. His mother, Dubba, worked hard for those children. She'd leave home in the morning and return late at night. She did whatever it took to keep a roof over their heads and rice and peas and chicken on the Sunday table. Then one night Dubba returned home late from work to find social service workers standing outside her door. A nosy neighbor had told the authorities that she was leaving Robbie and his siblings all alone. The state removed all the children. Robbie was sent to live with a foster family in Columbia. He pined for his mother. He cried every day. Finally, Dubba convinced the social workers she wasn't a bad mother and deserved to get her children back. Robbie always talked about the day he came home to Cloverdale. That house on Armstrong Street looked like a palace.

Robbie was great with his hands. He could cut hair. He left home and attended Denmark Tech in Bamberg, the same school that had trained Cliff and thousands of black barbers and beauticians. Robbie came home proud with his barber license. He framed it and hung it on the wall right over his station. Then, just like that, Robbie left home. Cloverdale couldn't hold him anymore. Robbie had to get out, to see the world, to explore his talents, to be himself. No more living a lie, pretending to be someone he wasn't. His mother understood. She never tried to hold him back.

Carolyn Brown reminisced about the first time she met Robbie. She couldn't forget his big grin and pirate earrings. Brown and her husband, Howard, and former high school friends left Charleston for college and founded Voices of Deliverance when they came back home to live, raise families, and sing. Robbie toured the world with Voices. But AIDS intervened. In late 2008 the group was preparing to fly to Paris without him.

Tricia Ann rose to deliver the eulogy. She spoke of the woman caught in adultery. Her accusers stood ready to condemn her to death by stoning. "Let him who is without sin cast the first stone." No one stepped forward.

There's a better day coming by and by when we reach that city in the sky.

As Tricia Ann spoke, one of Robbie's brothers stepped up to the casket. He ran his hands along the rail of the Carolina blue coffin. He paused, not saying a word, until a woman, maybe his wife or sister, walked up to him and placed an arm on his shoulder and led him back to his seat.

"Where are thine accusers?" Tricia Ann Starr preached. That was the scripture that came to her as soon as she got word of Robbie's death. "I know that we all judge."

Even though the woman of the Bible story had been found guilty under the law and could be put death, Jesus showed compassion for her.

"You have to stand before God for yourself," Tricia Ann told mourners. "No matter what she did, she was left alone to deal with her wrong." This message was not for Robbie. It was for those who knew his lifestyle and condemned him.

"You need to know the day will come when you will be left alone with God," she intoned. "You have to face God for yourself. What will your answer be?" Robbie lived two lives. He was openly gay in Charleston, where he shared an apartment with his male lover. In Clover, Robbie lived in the closet. Both halves of his life came together in that church that gray Saturday afternoon. He didn't live in Clover. He didn't want to die in Clover. He just wanted to be buried there near his mother, Dubba. She had died almost eight years before and was buried on a December day just like this. The last time Robbie spent more than a few days in Clover was when he came to care for her in 2000. He left his music, his plays, his singing, and his acting roles to be by his mother's side. He was the dutiful oldest son of Dubba, the woman who sold sweet potato pie and fried bread to her neighbors in Cloverdale. They called her the Candy Lady.

On Tricia Ann's twentieth anniversary she and Larry had visited Robbie in Charleston. Robbie showed them around the city and took them to Kiawah Island, where he sang with a jazz band. That night everyone seemed to love Robbie, and he reveled in it. That adulation seemed so different from the disrespect and hostility he received back in his Cloverdale neighborhood.

Charleston was a world away from Clover, like separate continents culturally.

Robbie excelled in musicals. When he climbed on stage his personality changed—all his inhibitions dissolved, regrets faded under the glow of his transformation. He sang like Donny Hathaway reincarnated.

When Tricia Ann and Larry walked into Robbie's apartment, they sensed someone else was there but out of sight. Robbie instinctively hid his lover for fear that his small-town visitors would condemn his decadent big-city lifestyle. But he didn't need to hide from Tricia Ann and Larry. They had always known, all those years. How he hung around with a certain group of guys. He didn't run with the hoodlums and gangbangers. But this was still Robbie.

"Don't do that," Tricia Ann admonished him. "I'm not God. I'm not here to judge you. This is your house. What you do is your business." Those words liberated Robbie. He relaxed and smiled and introduced them to his friend. Those days Robbie still looked lean and strong. But when he came home in 2000 to care for his mother, frailty clung to his frame like the first dust of a dry, parched summer. The skin on his round face seemed taut. His round brown eyes orbited more prominently in their sockets. Robbie seemed to wear the same gown of illnesses that had stalked Clover for a decade. Formerly strong young men and women faded away in plain sight amid a cruel mixture of silence and denial.

Dubba required dialysis. Robbie rode with her back and forth to Rock Hill. Robbie made her laugh. He nagged her until she ate. He met her every need. He was the dutiful oldest son.

Lesions appeared on his face and marred his good looks. At his mother's funeral, Robbie tried to sing her favorite song, "Amazing Grace." He couldn't finish it. It might have been just grief, but it sounded like shortness of breath. He was ill that day. Even before the service started, he went back to the kitchen. Tricia Ann followed him.

"Are you OK?"

"I have to try. Momma wanted me to try," he sobbed. "People are gonna know."

"You could tell he was sick. That day he was shaking," she says. "It was not just grief; it was his body."

He wore a black suit and white shirt. Neither fit right.

"*I once was lost but now I'm found.*" Then his voice broke. He tried to play it off.

"I can't finish," he announced and walked back to the kitchen. His friends followed him back. After the service, his younger siblings had questions.

"Something was wrong with my brother," said James Lamey.

"They always figured I knew what was wrong with Robbie," Tricia Ann says. "They'd say, 'Something is wrong with our brother, and you know what it is.' I said, 'He was upset,'" Tricia Ann recalled.

But even as his mother died, Robbie knew he had begun his death march. After Dubba was gone, he lingered in Clover for a few weeks afterward to settle her affairs. He and Tricia Ann rode back and forth to the county seat in York. Robbie talked about what his mother had endured— his childhood, her sacrifices, when she lost them to foster care because she couldn't afford a babysitter. Dubba tried to be a good mother. She worked for them. Robbie thanked Tricia Ann for taking care of her.

He looked forward to going back to the Low Country. But he carried a burden. He was living with AIDS, and he hadn't told his siblings. How could he? He was somewhat successful; he had a career. That would have let them down. He would be disappointing them. He didn't want them to look at him differently.

The Monday morning after his mother's funeral, Tricia Ann saw Robbie walking toward her house. His steps were unsteady.

"Did you take your meds?" she asked.

"No. They make me sick." Robbie wore his favorite blue jogging suit. In his hand he held an envelope and a cassette tape bound with brown rubber bands.

"I want you to give this to my brother after I leave," he said, as he gave Tricia Ann the envelope and the tape. He sat down on the couch the way people do before a long, heartfelt conversation. He talked about trying to put his mother's affairs in order.

"I want you to do me a favor." He pulled out a hand-addressed envelope.

"What's that?" she asked. It was a letter.

"Give it to my family after I'm gone."

"Why?"

"Read it."

Slowly she opened the unsealed envelope. The letter was written in neat, stylish cursive, the penmanship of someone who wrote with care and pain.

To my brothers and sisters:

I wish there were some way I could tell you this. I am HIV positive. I have AIDS. I am sorry. I never meant to shame you. I am your older brother. You look up to me. I didn't want you to be put in the position of having to defend me. I am sorry.

She placed the cassette in the player. Robbie spoke in a clear voice, then he began to sob, his voice filled with pain, shame, hurt, betrayal, the despair of a brother telling his siblings that he was going to die. That was bad enough. Worse was that he felt so ashamed that he couldn't bear to tell them face-to-face. "I'm sorry for all the pain I caused you. I am sorry that I have left you to fight my battles on the street. I never meant to cause you pain. I'm sorry. I'm sorry."

His living will was wrapped in elastic bands and shame. He asked Tricia Ann to deliver the letter and tape once he was safely back home in open-minded, nonjudgmental Charleston. He sat quietly and watched her as she read and reread the words. They opened a floodgate of emotion. She cried. She cried out of sadness. Sadness that Robbie's secrets were so deep and dark that he couldn't tell his brothers and his sisters. Sadness for his shame, shame for his lifestyle as a gay man, shame that his actions would one day bring the burden of death and stigma on his family. Tears rolled down her face.

"I knew the outcome of his life," she says. She tried to encourage him to fight. The letter sounded as if he were giving up. The medicines made him feel bad. She tried to assure him that he was going to have better days. She struggled to find the right words to encourage him. She tried to invoke Dubba's spirit to save her son.

"What would she be saying to you right now?" she asked. His mother knew about Robbie's AIDS before she died. He told her. She knew about his life. Mothers always know. "She didn't judge him. She loved him. He loved her."

Tricia Ann is not one for tears. They hamper her ability to do her job. But that morning as she sat with Robbie, she wept bitterly, uncontrollably. And when she regained her composure or some semblance of it, she became angry.

"This is a coward's way out. I will not do it." Her defiant words belied the sentiments of her heart. She knew she would do as he asked. "OK, I'll do it. When are you leaving?"

"In a couple of days."

Robbie called to say he had reached home safely. But he hadn't changed his mind. He wanted her to give his siblings the package.

Tricia struggled with her assignment. The package sat on her night-stand for days. Days turned into weeks. Each day she looked at it, her reluctance multiplied. She hoped that Robbie would call back and say he had changed his mind. As the days and weeks passed, she knew the phone call from Charleston would never come. So she stalled and prayed for time— the right time. The New Year wasn't the right time. The sisters and brothers had just lost their mother; Tricia Ann couldn't drop a second bombshell. Announcing that Robbie had AIDS would feel like a second death in the family. His siblings should have known. They should have guessed that athletic, suave, strong Robbie had been replaced by a shrunken, withered man whose voice no longer danced over the words he spoke, whose vocal cords no longer cleared the wax in their ears.

And so as America prepared to inaugurate George W. Bush, the first president in the new millennium, Tricia Ann walked around with a private preoccupation. This was a strange situation. This wasn't her guilt. This wasn't her shame.

Soon afterward, Robbie started feeling better. He was upbeat. He returned to work. He was back singing. One day early in 2001, he called Tricia Ann.

"Have you given the family the letter?" he asked.

"No," she said. "I thought you would have called me to tell me you had changed your mind. I'm not ready to give it to them."

He said, "Give it to them."

Finally she couldn't bear to see that envelope and cassette tape a moment longer. She called Robbie's younger brother. Tricia Ann walked into her bedroom and retrieved the envelope and the cassette tape bound tightly together with a brown rubber band. When Tricia Ann gave the package to James, he said he knew. He started reading the letter. He shook his head.

"I suspected it. In my guts I knew all along," he said to me after Robbie's funeral.

"All those pills he's been taking, that sickly look. I've been in Clover long enough to know that look, especially when it's my own brother."

Soon afterward, James called. He told Robbie he loved him. "Why didn't you tell me that yourself? Why did you feel you couldn't tell me to my face? We are brothers; it don't matter," he told him. "I'm not ashamed of you. You are my brother."

James recalled that conversation the cold December afternoon after the funeral. Unlike the reedlike Robbie, James was built like a linebacker: powerful shoulders, tank-like midsection, tree-trunk arms, and a thick neck that held up a clean-shaven head. James had lost one arm above the elbow when he got sucked into a conveyor belt in 1988. Dressed in his dark suit, James dressed the abbreviated arm in a black sock, like a baby truncheon ready to punish evildoers.

James had stared death in the face and lived. He loved his brother. Nothing his brother said or did would change that.

"Do your brothers and sisters know?" I asked.

"No. Or if they do, they haven't mentioned it. You know how people are afraid of the AIDS."

A year after his mother's death, even as America tried to regain its bearings following the terrorist attacks of September 11, 2001, James was in a celebratory mood. He was finally getting married. He had grown children ready to start families of their own. He wanted to walk down the aisle. He wanted his brother to serenade him.

James called Robbie. Over the long-distance telephone line, James thought Robbie didn't sound like himself. He seemed distracted, forgetful even. James was forced to repeat the details of his upcoming nuptials.

He wanted Robbie to sing at the wedding. "Sure, just come and get me."

Robbie couldn't drive.

James drove three hours down Interstate 77 and then cut southeast on I-26 to Charleston. When he arrived, Robbie looked in no shape to travel. He wandered around the apartment trying to collect his things. But mostly, he fussed about the pills. He panicked about not having enough for a short visit to Clover.

At home, each morning, James watched as his brother consumed a pharmacist's supply cabinet's worth of green pills, white pills, and capsules. He gulped each down with a hard, swooshing swallow.

"What's the matter with you?"

"I'm sick."

Finally, the day before the wedding, during the rehearsal, Robbie walked outside where he found the mother of the bride. He started talking openly for the first time. It seemed as if he needed to unload the terrible, secret burden he had long carried.

"I am HIV positive. I have full-blown AIDS. I'm not sure how much time I have left."

It would be another seven years before Tricia Ann and James would finally get the call.

Paramedics rushed Robbie to Roper Hospital. He'd had a massive stroke. That was Friday. The siblings drove down to Charleston on Sunday to see Robbie. He was in pretty bad shape. That night after they left the hospital, he took a turn for the worse. There was bleeding on the brain, swelling. The doctor called James. "Do you want us to put him on life support?"

James said yes, but he asked his pastor, Tricia Ann, anyway. She thought that was unnecessary. She counseled against putting Robbie on life support. "That's not what Robbie would have wanted."

The siblings talked. On Monday they called the doctor. Robbie's blood pressure was dropping.

"Do you want to take him off life support?" This time the siblings didn't hesitate. Yes.

The doctor called a nurse as a witness.

The family prepared to drive down to say a final good-bye. They were getting ready to leave at 1:15 PM when the doctor called back. Robert was gone. He was forty-nine.

His siblings called Tricia Ann in a panic. "What do we do?" one of them asked.

"You can go down if you want to, but he's gone. There's nothing you can do." They had two choices. They could bring Robbie home for burial or leave him in Charleston and have the ceremony down there. "If you are bringing him home, there's no point in going down there," Tricia Ann told James.

They decided to bring him home to Clover for a December funeral, just like the one they'd had for their mother eight years before. Robbie wasn't buried next to his mother, though. Robbie was a pauper. A black man living with AIDS often dies without life insurance. Family members must scrounge for scarce dollars to pay for a modest funeral.

Death deals strictly in cash, not credit. After the funeral services, even as the mourners sat in the kitchen eating fried chicken, stuffing, macaroni and cheese, corn on the cob, and peach cobbler, Robbie's brother, now the head of the family, pulled a wad of twenties out of his wallet and handed them to the funeral director. As the mourners ate, a black hearse drove from Mount Carmel Road on the way to the burial ground. The vehicle passed the majestic, stately colonial houses, their windows adorned with green wreaths and red bows for the coming Christmas holidays, a marked contrast to the gray austere sky and the grim task that lay ahead of the grave digger.

Minutes later a solitary vehicle pulled into Armstrong Street—where Robbie grew up—and parked at the cemetery. No entourage trailed behind. When the Generation Funeral Home hearse loaded Robbie's body and drove to the black cemetery in Clover, his fellow choir members stayed behind at the church, eating macaroni and cheese and fried chicken with all the other mourners. Then they climbed into their van and headed back to Charleston.

No one stood to throw flowers on Robbie's coffin. By sundown, Robbie rested under a mound of damp clay; two large floral decorations made up of lilies and carnations sat atop the freshly turned mound. The cemetery sits on a low ridge that looks west toward the Great Smoky Mountains on the North Carolina-Tennessee border, toward freedom, the wild.

After Tricia Ann preached the eulogy at Robbie's funeral, after all the food was shared and the mourners from Charleston with their red bows on their lapels had climbed into their white van and headed home to the Low Country, the pastor of True Word of God Fire Baptized Holiness Church allowed herself a break to sit on the front pews of the now-empty sanctuary next to the kerosene heater.

Then her cell phone rang.

It was Barbara Dixon, a church member and longtime friend. Her words hung with concern. It was about Girard. As she spoke, the weight of the news made Tricia Ann's shoulders sag. She had begun that morning attending the funeral in neighboring Gastonia, North Carolina, for a cousin who had succumbed to cancer at age forty-three. After the songs and speeches and cold clay on a casket, she drove forty minutes back to Clover, then to her church in York to officiate at Robbie's funeral at midday.

Barbara sounded hysterical. The doctor at Piedmont Medical Center had sent Girard home under the care of hospice. Girard, her baby brother, was coming home to die. Within minutes, an ambulance drove west from Rock Hill, its siren silent. No amount of haste could help the patient inside that Saturday evening.

Within a week, flowers would decorate Girard's grave a few feet away from Robbie's.

25

GIRARD

On Saturday, December 6, 2008, an ambulance pulled up to the red brick house at 303 Kings Mountain Street. The paramedics wheeled Girard on the gurney up the slight wooden incline of a recently constructed ramp. Tricia Ann's brother John had built the ramp for Barbara so she wouldn't have to struggle to lift Girard out of the wheelchair and carry him up the front steps whenever she shuttled him back and forth from dialysis.

Girard had returned to Piedmont Medical Center in Rock Hill just days after the hospital had released him following a two-month stay. Now, on that cold, gray December evening, he made his final trip home. As Tricia Ann ended the phone call from Barbara, her thoughts immediately turned to Girard's siblings, who had little experience dealing with death. When Girard died, they were going to need an experienced hand.

So that night, after she left the empty church, Tricia Ann drove home, then circled by the Clover Community Cemetery to see where Robbie was buried. On a warmer day she could have walked from home to the cemetery and then to Girard's house just north of the invisible line that separated white and black Clover. Girard's one-story brick ranch sat on the white side of the line. That was just like Girard—breaking the rules, flouting convention, like the well-groomed dreadlocks he wore to work at Bank of America, like driving with his convertible top down even after winter arrived, like admitting to those who asked and those who didn't that he was gay.

That evening, I accompanied Tricia Ann as she walked into Girard's home, with its high, majestic ceiling and burnished wood floor. We walked up the wheelchair ramp to the front door. As we entered the living room, the gaiety and merriment of the Christmas lights next door seemed to mock the solemnity of the proceedings inside. A decorated Christmas tree stood in the living room, a testament to someone's desperate need to acknowledge the joyous season despite the sad reality lying in the hospital bed twenty feet away. Tricia Ann walked into the bedroom where Girard lay on white hospital linen, covered by two blankets. His jet-black dreadlocks splashed like a horse's mane against the white cotton pillows.

His blanket covered him up to his neck. One arm stuck out from under the covers, exposing a skinny wrist adorned by two hospital-issue wristbands. Girard's skin looked dark and taut. His eyes were mostly closed, but when he opened them, they seemed sunken in their sockets as they rolled back, exposing only the whites as if he were about to die. His breathing was labored and shallow. Tricia Ann called his name.

"Gee." He weakly turned his head toward her, his eyes opening slowly into blotchy white slits. He opened his mouth. No words. To the inexpert observer it was unclear if Girard was awake or asleep, conscious or comatose. His oldest sister stood beside the bed looking at him helplessly.

The room was furnished in a stark but elegant style. African art hung on the walls. Small cabinets stood stocked with cologne. Girard loved to smell good. He embarked on shopping trips to Macy's to buy nothing but colognes. He thought nothing of spending $200 on a five-ounce bottle of Ralph Lauren. Bottles, one for every occasion, filled the shelves in the bathroom cabinets.

Girard was single, indulgent but generous. He loved his sisters and their children. He also loved men. He never apologized. He never felt the urge to.

When does a boy discover that he loves boys instead of girls, and how does he live his life knowing that desire, choice, or fate could shorten his lifespan?

William Girard Lindsay was born on Friday, November 1, 1968, as Americans prepared to elect Richard Nixon president. Like Carolyn, Girard was the baby of the bunch. His mother, Thomasine Lindsay, had three girls and three boys. The Lindsay family lived in a small shack on what is now a vacant spit of grass just a stone's throw from the town's black burial grounds. From their front yard, Girard and his siblings could sing along with the mourners who accompanied the dead. They were close enough to hear the shovel hit the hard clay as the grave diggers prepared for another burial.

Girard and his siblings earned a reputation for being poor but proud. They struggled to make ends meet like their neighbors, but the children carried themselves with a regal deportment that belied their lowly station. During picnics and cookouts, most families played touch football or volleyball or tossed horseshoes. But the Lindsays were different. They played badminton and croquet.

Thomasine, like many of her Clover neighbors, worked long hours in the textile mills, first at Marion Yarns, then at the American Thread Company, until crippling arthritis and gout curtailed her work life. Surgeons replaced both hips and both kneecaps, but Barbara, her middle daughter, remembers that the surgeries only seemed to make her mother worse. When Barbara was about twelve years old and Girard was about six, friction from living in their grandmother's overcrowded home prompted the family to move out of the house on Armstrong Street into a Clover Public Housing Authority apartment in the projects on Pinkney Street.

The family survived on meager welfare payments—Thomasine's disability check and help from social services. Eventually the two older siblings went to work. By pooling the paychecks and welfare, the family lived comfortably enough. Barbara remembers that, unlike some of her neighbors, who only ate meat on Sundays, the Lindsays ate three meals a day and always had meat on their dinner plate.

Although Barbara didn't know it at the time, the trajectory of Girard's life was altered during those crucial early years. A married man who had children of his own accosted Girard one night as he was walking along a path behind the apartments and raped him. Girard was nine or ten years old. After that, Girard tried to avoid his molester, but the man always found opportunities to intercept and molest the youngster. No one in his family knew the story until Girard finally broke down and told Barbara in the last few years of his life. "He would catch him by himself," Barbara says.

Later, abuse grew into seduction and seduction into a permanent long-term relationship, in which the molested turned to his abuser for love and comfort. "That was all he knew," Barbara said. "He could have confronted him, but he didn't." That relationship continued for years until Girard was grown and in college. He found other loves but always found a way to be with the man who first molested him. Eventually the man died of AIDS. But that was later.

Meanwhile, even as his mother became sicker and his sexual confusion spiraled, Girard excelled in the classroom. His Clover High schoolmates remember him well. Following Girard's death in December 2008, an e-mail went out from the Clover High School Reunion website alerting former classmates. No one needed any reminder of who Girard was—they remembered the flamboyant classmate with the flashy hair.

When Girard graduated from high school in 1986, Barb and her siblings threw him the biggest party in Cloverdale that year. It was supposed to be his splashy send-off to college. But with his mother's illness, money was hard to come by, and it took Girard a year to secure enough grants and financial aid to pay for Winthrop University. In the fall of 1987, he moved his things into the university dorms. But twenty-five miles couldn't separate him and Barb. After she finished working second shift, she punched her time card and drove to Rock Hill. She slept many nights in Girard's college dorm and then drove home the next morning. "We went to college together," she says.

Girard dreamed of teaching. While attending Winthrop, he taught courses on how to work on websites. He always talked about working hard and retiring early so he could travel. He was determined to get out of Clover. At one point he even moved to Charlotte, where he lived with a white lover for a while. He moved back to Clover soon after a burglar broke into his apartment. Afterward, he talked incessantly about moving to a bigger city. "Had he lived, he would have moved to Atlanta," Tricia Ann says. "Clover was too small for him."

Traditionally, two kinds of black gay men lived in Clover: those whose lives were defined by their sexual preference and those whose lives were spent trying to hide or deny their sexual identity. Girard refused to be either. He cut his own path.

He was a flamboyantly gay, college-educated, corporate black man. He wasn't ashamed of it. Girard frequented the bathhouses and gay bars in the big city. He traveled frequently. He had a life outside Clover. His suits and colognes and cars, his education and job, set him apart from many of the black men and women with whom he grew up. "He lived his life. He enjoyed his life," Tricia Ann says.

Girard spoke most eloquently through his hair. Sometimes it was a jet-black perm; later, blond or black dreadlocks framed his dark brown, narrow face and high cheekbones. At Barb's wedding, the bride wore an ivory gown, while Girard chose an all-white tuxedo with green cummerbund and vest and white shoes. He was neither best man nor giving away the bride; he was just the guy who sang the solo. But it didn't matter to Girard. No husband could ever get between him and his favorite sister.

When her mother died, Barb moved out and took Girard with her. She treated him like the son she never had. She fussed over him. She took care of him. She mothered him.

After Winthrop, he worked in a series of banking jobs. Banks are known for their conservative, corporate culture, but that didn't deter Girard. He was comfortable and competent. "Girard took pride in everything he did," Tricia Ann says.

He worked for BB&T and then, later, Bank of America. By 2006 he had been promoted to assistant vice president for change. The desktop name plaque with his title is displayed on the entertainment center of his sister's house. His LinkedIn page stands as an everlasting memorial to his corporate efficiency and the ambition of an upwardly mobile black man.

When he got home from work, Girard excelled in the kitchen. He watched the Food Network for hours on his high-definition flat screen TV. He loved to cook and entertain. There was nothing he wouldn't try. When he moved into the house on Kings Mountain Street, he loved nothing better than to cook for his siblings and their children.

So when in 1997 he learned he was infected with HIV, Girard didn't tell Barb or anyone else. "He was afraid they wouldn't eat his food," Tricia Ann says.

Girard caught the flu. A year after the panic Cliff's list of names unleashed in 1996, Girard, the smart, responsible guy who had it all together, was diagnosed with full-blown AIDS when his kidneys failed.

Girard didn't tell Tricia Ann he was HIV positive, but after that first serious illness, she knew right away. He kept insisting it was kidney failure, but he couldn't fool her. Even after Tricia Ann confronted him, Girard steadfastly refused to tell any of his siblings that he had developed acquired immune deficiency syndrome.

All along Barb wondered about her brother's failing health. "Being around my pastor, seeing AIDS patients and their transformation," she says. "You can see the skin tone change."

When Girard got sick, Barbara confronted him. "Do you have AIDS?" she asked, her voice saturated with worry.

"No, I don't. It's just that my kidneys shut down."

"I let it go," she says. Barb sang farewell to Nita and to others who died of AIDS. She witnessed the suffering of Carolyn and Tracy up close. She knew what AIDS did to people she loved. It was understandable that she let herself believe that her brother, the one person she loved more than any other, didn't have that dreaded illness.

And for the next eleven years, he stuck with that story: he suffered from kidney failure. It was the joke around the neighborhood. He battled a litany of AIDS-related illnesses: staph infections, kidney infections, lesions, blisters, pneumonia.

AIDS weakens the body quickly and brings the person down. Each time, Girard bounced back. He didn't let it stop him. He quietly tried to encourage Tracy and Lawrence, a former classmate and neighbor, to take their meds. Lawrence (name changed), Tricia Ann's relative by marriage, had AIDS. His relatives fought to keep his secret. For a while Lawrence sought treatment at a private clinic in Charlotte, but when the money and the meds ran out, he steadfastly refused to go to the Christopher Clinic, which might have extended his life. When he died in September 2003, Girard's poetry graced Lawrence's funeral program.

By 2004, protease inhibitors were transforming AIDS and HIV into something more closely resembling a chronic illness, nothing like the death sentence it was for many of Lawrence and Girard's neighbors. But for those like Lawrence and Girard, the desire to keep their illness secret and the shame of it all was too much.

"So many times he wanted to go and tell people who were HIV positive: 'You can live a normal life by taking the medicine, if you did what you were supposed to do,'" Tricia Ann says. But Girard feared that if he became a cheerleader for taking your AIDS medicine, he would be marked as a person with AIDS. "He didn't want to be judged," Tricia Ann says. "He wanted to be Girard, the young black man who had it going on." Maybe that was selfish of Girard. If you can help someone else, why not? But the equation of shame is not so simple.

As Tracy gave up, Girard tried to talk to her, to tell her that there was hope, even with AIDS. He wrote songs to encourage himself and his friends. "I Live a Life of Desperation" was Girard's song, his way of saying without saying what he was going through. Each year for pastor appreciation day, he sang Tricia Ann a song.

After his first bout of kidney failure in 1997, Girard returned to church. For a while, he tried to renounce his gay lifestyle. He and Tricia Ann talked long into the night about what it meant for one man to love another. He gave her a tour of gay Charlotte nightlife. He showed her the gay clubs and bathhouses where he used to go.

"I was curious," Tricia Ann confessed. "I wanted to ask the question, how was it kissing a man?"

Girard answered without hesitation by simply rephrasing her question. "How does a man kiss a woman?"

The final year of Girard's life started well. He had begun to work from home. He owned a time-share and loved the beach. He planned a beach vacation. He was worried about Barb and all the energy she spent caring for him. "He felt guilty that she was spending so much of her time with him," Tricia Ann says.

On Mother's Day 2008 catastrophe struck. Barb blamed the bats that inhabited the attic in Girard's house. He was so afraid of the flying creatures that one night he fled his house barefoot and walked over to Barb's to ask his brother-in-law to come and kill the bat that was flying inside the house. That Sunday night Girard called for help. He was trying to kill a bat in his bedroom when he fell and hurt his leg. He couldn't get up. When Barb reached the house, she couldn't get in. All the doors were locked. Eventually, she and her husband broke in through Girard's bedroom window. She called 911. When the paramedics arrived, they thought Girard had sprained his leg so they treated him and left. The next morning, Girard couldn't stand. He couldn't put any pressure on his leg. Barb called 911 at 1:00 PM, but the paramedics didn't show up for seven hours. When Girard arrived at Piedmont Medical Center that night, the waiting room was so crowded patients were lined up against the wall. Girard screamed in agony.

"He kept asking for something for the pain," she recalls. X-rays showed Girard suffered a broken fibula. It took months before Girard could move without pain. He used a walker and by mid-August had graduated to using a cane. "He was happy and excited. He wanted fried chicken and corn," Barb says.

No sooner than Girard had recovered from his broken leg than other complications developed. Late summer 2008, while undergoing home peritoneal dialysis for kidney failure, he had a "bad exchange." Barbara thought a bag of dialysate that was put into Girard's peritoneal cavity to help drain waste from his body was tainted. That infection sent Girard back to Piedmont Medical Center, where he spent much of October and November, including his birthday. Girard turned forty on November 1. His friends brought ice cream cake and balloons and a plaque to his hospital room. The plaque read HAPPY BIRTHDAY, GEE.

It was signed with his friends' names and inscribed with Girard's favorite Bible verse: Job 14:14: "If a man dies, shall he live again? All the days of my appointed time will I wait, till my change come."

When Tricia Ann saw him during that time, Girard's appearance had changed drastically. He had begun to take on that ashy look Carolyn once feared. She sensed the end was not far off.

But Girard still hadn't told his beloved sister what was killing him. He was convinced that if he told Barbara it would devastate her. "He felt he had let her down," Tricia Ann says. "His thing was making his family proud."

And so as the leaves turned yellow, then orange, as nature acknowledged the coming winter in the Piedmont region, Girard finally resolved to tell his sister the truth. She could bathe him, clean him, and change his clothes like a baby, but he still hadn't told her the truth. He told Tricia Ann that he wanted Dr. Craig Charles, his infectious disease physician, to talk to Barb. She deserved to know. After all, she had neglected her daughter and husband to spend every waking hour with him at the hospital. But even as he waited for the right time to make his request, fate intervened.

One day while Barb was sitting in the room with Girard, a nurse walked in. She wanted to talk to him about his condition.

"Do you know how you got AIDS?" the nurse asked.

"Yes."

After the nurse left, Girard lay there while Barb waited for him to say something. When he didn't, she spoke up. "When were you gonna tell me?" she asked.

"I wanted to tell you all along," he said. "Are you disappointed in me?"

"No, I'm not disappointed. I'm hurt . . . hurt that you felt you had to go through this by yourself." That was Girard's biggest hurdle in having AIDS. He had lived his life as a beacon, an example of accomplishment for his siblings and his nieces and nephews. How could Girard admit that he had been careless enough, weak enough, to contract the same disease that had killed dozens of the drug addicts and promiscuous men and women who walked his neighborhood streets? He was supposed to be better than that. AIDS undermined Girard's sense of superiority. But as Thanksgiving came and went and the Christmas season beckoned, Girard and his friends and relatives were forced to confront the consequences.

———— ⌘ ————

On Sunday, December 7, 2008, the morning after Girard came home from the hospital for the last time, the morning after Robbie's battered body found a home below the Carolina sod, Tricia Ann climbed into her car and drove to church. On her way, she pulled up in front of Girard's house and walked up the ramp to see him. Girard's fellow church members surrounded his bed and tried to offer spiritual comfort. He used to attend Tricia Ann's True Word of God Fire Baptized Holiness Church but had left a few years earlier to join another congregation. He still considered Tricia Ann his personal pastor. "I'm leaving the church; I'm not leaving you," he used to tell her. Implicit in his words: she would officiate at his funeral and eulogize him.

After church, before she went to work that Sunday afternoon, Tricia Ann stopped by for an hour to see how Girard was doing. She tried to comfort Barb and went in to check on Girard. When Tricia Ann walked in to see the patient, she was amazed at how much he had deteriorated in twenty-four hours. She knew his end drew near. It wouldn't be weeks or days but hours. Tonight would be the night, she thought. Shaken by what she saw, Tricia Ann stepped outside to the back porch to compose herself.

"What's wrong?" Barb asked.

"He's turned ashy," Tricia Ann said. "Carolyn didn't want to be ashy." Tricia Ann had sensed the death angel loitering in the room, waiting for Girard's golden hour, but she didn't tell Barb what she was thinking. She tried to encourage her. "Stay close and be strong," she told her. "Say your good-byes."

"Is he going to leave us?" she asked.

"It won't be long," Tricia Ann replied, then drove to her job at a local fast-food restaurant. On Sunday nights, she finished work around eleven. When she arrived at the house, one of Girard's sisters was trying to change him. She struggled with his weight. She was trying to lift him by herself. Tricia Ann removed her coat and apron to give the woman a hand. Those on death's door need careful and compassionate handling.

For the uninitiated, it's a messy chore. But for the experienced, it is a methodical exercise. Tricia Ann cleaned Girard and changed his white bed linen, then prepared for a long night. She busied herself, straightening up the room while some of Girard's relatives stood around the bed and talked. Then Girard opened his eyes.

"I love you," Tricia Ann said looking at him. "I'm mad at you." He reached out his hand so she could hold him. She smiled at him, and he looked at her. Although Girard's mouth remained shut tight, he seemed to be telling her something—that he loved her too and that he was sorry for the pain he was causing. Then he began to inhale deeply and groaned.

"Do you want something for the pain?" she asked. He batted his eyes in response. She gave him drops of sedative on his tongue. "He's going to rest now," she told Barb. "You can take a break."

Around 4:00 AM Monday, December 8, 2008, Tricia Ann was startled by the sound of Girard's breathing; he took short, abbreviated breaths. As she stood next to the bed, he turned his head toward the door. She walked around to the other side of the bed so he could see her face, so he would know that someone was there. She rubbed his hand and his head and talked to him.

"It's OK to be with the Lord," she said, and then walked out of the room to fetch Barb. By the time they returned, Girard's eyes were closed and a sense of peace enveloped the room. But the quiet was quickly shattered as Barb saw her brother's lifeless body. She had wanted to be there.

"He didn't want anyone to be there," Tricia Ann says. "God granted his wish to leave without the family being there."

"I don't think she could have taken it. Watching a sister or brother die is painful," she said. "When you are dealing with someone you love, it's not easy."

EPILOGUE

December 2008 was a month of tears. Just weeks after Tricia Ann buried Robbie and Girard, she stood over another casket. William, a brother born fourteen months earlier than her, the brother who had survived a gunshot in 1979, was dead.

After his mother's death, William migrated north like many black South Carolinians. He settled in New Jersey, married, and raised a family. Now William was gone. He was barely fifty. The third of Ann Mae's children had come to join her early in the family plot at the St. James Methodist Church cemetery. Tricia Ann's grandfather had helped build the church, and as payment, his family and descendants were given land near the church cemetery to bury their dead.

And Annie Mae's children and descendants wasted no time trying to fill up the burial ground. The headstones are granite monuments to the hurt of the past few decades. Annie Mae's headstone stands modestly next to Tracy's with a space in between. Near Annie Mae is a flat stone that marks Carolyn's resting place. Her brother, Robert "Woody," who died in 1997 while Carolyn was serving time, rests nearby. John, the oldest sibling, has reserved the space between Tracy and Annie Mae. Next to Annie Mae lies her delinquent husband, Samuel. Although they were separated for years, the two never divorced. He who had abandoned his family in life rejoined them in death. The family has dwindled down to Tricia Ann, Betty (the sister who was adopted by relatives), John, and Danny, a brother who lives in Rock Hill. A third brother, Spanky, is serving a life term behind bars.

The testimony to the dying was just as poignant in the Clover Community Cemetery, where the town's black citizens lay their dead. Robbie sleeps a few feet away from Girard. Between them lies Nanette, a young mother who died just months before the two men. She was a friend of theirs. Up and down the rows of headstones, the graves tell short stories about the short lives of those who died. Brevity makes for unanswered questions.

With posterity lies the task of speculating about who and what they were and why they died so young.

Less than an hour away in Rock Hill, Linda Ashley spends her days at Winthrop University. She's the director of field instruction and continuing education in the department of social work. In that role, she trains students who plan to do what she used to do. One twist is that now she sends undergraduate social work interns to the Christopher Clinic to learn the craft she once practiced.

If you called the Christopher Clinic on a Wednesday or Thursday, Chris Blanton would be likely to answer the phone. The former ombudsman works part time as a receptionist at the clinic named in his honor. As the agency prepared to celebrate its tenth anniversary in fall 2010, employees were packing boxes. After a decade in its nondescript office building on Camden Avenue, the clinic found a new, larger home in an office park. With a staff of several dozen employees, the agency has become part of what Washington, DC, ACT UP cofounder Wayne Turner once called "AIDS Inc."

The Health Resources Services Administration website shows that in 2010, Catawba Care, as the organization is now called, received $576,711 in Ryan White program funds for outpatient early intervention services, plus another $58,000 development planning grant. The emphasis of the Ryan White CARE Act has shifted from dying to living. Given the effectiveness of modern antiretroviral cocktails, money goes toward medical care and creating access to medical care and early intervention—getting those who test HIV positive to begin medications as soon as possible to delay or avoid the onset of full-blown AIDS.

Some of the people with AIDS who came to the clinic when it first opened still do. They are among the 450 people who come for care. Of those, 302, or 68 percent, of them have an undetectable viral load. That doesn't mean they no longer test positive for HIV. They could still pass on the virus through unprotected sex. The virus is just not growing in their bodies. It's not active. "It means that the battle is at a standoff," says Catawba Care director Anita Case. That kind of prognosis would have been impossible three decades ago.

While there is still no proven cure for AIDS, better medicines help people live longer. However, those meds aren't always available because people live too far away from a place like the Christopher Clinic, have no health insurance, or live in a state with long waiting lists because their legislatures have slashed AIDS Drug Assistance Program budgets. With the recession that began in 2008, many states cut back on AIDS funding. And southern states such as South Carolina, known for their stingy health care funding even in good times, are usually the hardest hit. Thankfully, some pharmaceutical companies have stepped in to fill the need.

So with free and effective medications, why are people in small towns still dying of AIDS? No medicine can cure the shame that some people still bear from having the disease. Like an unwanted facial tattoo, that stain clings to them, keeps them quiet, always hiding in plain sight. For people with AIDS who live in small, southern, conservative, rural towns, their physical illness is only half their battle. Some patients use the back door of the Christopher Clinic to avoid being seen in the parking lot or lobby. Some refuse to come at all because they know someone who works at the clinic. "They spend more energy trying to avoid the truth, so they end up suffering because of that," says Dr. Charles, the clinic's medical director

That was Tracy and Girard's story, as it was with so many others. And those left behind struggle with the consequences. In the summer of 2010, I visited Barbara, the sister who loved Girard more than any lover could. It had been eighteen months since his death, but to her, Girard was still there. She sat on his couch. Her living room was furnished with the dark-colored furniture and tasteful accessories that had once decorated his living room. It all belonged to him. Now it was hers. She slept on the bed he used to sleep on. His music collection, a mixture of gospel and secular CDs, occupied a rack to the side of her living room. On the entertainment center above the TV sat a brown nameplate: W. GIRARD LINDSAY, ASSISTANT VICE PRESIDENT. Barbara can almost see Girard's headstone from her front door. She tries not to visit too often.

Barb and Tricia Ann still have long conversations. The pastor believes that her parishioner will never get over her brother as long as she keeps so many reminders of him so close to her. At some point she must let go and move on. After all, Tricia Ann has learned the art of letting go. When you lose those you've loved as much as she has, then letting go becomes like air. You exhale to survive. But Barbara was much less familiar with loss, with death. And so, a year and a half after Girard closed his eyes for the last time, he was still a raw subject in her Cloverdale household. Tears came easily. She talked about him in the present tense, as if his absence was merely a temporary inconvenience. As if he was still there. In a way, he kind of was; he always will be.

APPENDIX

AIDS ORGANIZATIONS IN THE SOUTH

PRIVATE AND NONPROFIT ORGANIZATIONS

ALABAMA

AIDS Alabama
3521 7th Avenue South
Birmingham, AL 35222
Phone: (205) 324-9822, ext. 25
www.aidsalabama.org

AIDS Action Coalition of Huntsville
P.O. Box 2409 / 35804
600 St. Clair Avenue, Building 6, Suite 14
Huntsville, AL 35801
Phone: (256) 536-4700 or (800) 728-3603
Fax: (256) 536-4117
www.aidsactioncoalition.org

Birmingham AIDS Outreach
P.O. Box 550070
Birmingham, AL 35255
205 32nd Street South #101
Birmingham, AL 35233
Phone: (205) 322-4197

Fax: (205) 322-2131
www.birminghamaidsoutreach.org

South Alabama CARES
2054 Dauphin Street
Mobile, AL 36606
Phone: (251) 471-5277 or (800) 758-7754
Fax: (251) 471-5294
www.masshelps.org

Selma AIR
P.O. Box 396
Selma, AL 36701
Phone: (334) 872-6795 or (800) 486-7591
Fax: (334) 872-3632

AIDS in Minorities
P.O. Box 1116
1925 Bessemer Road
Birmingham, AL 35208
Phone: (205) 781-1654

Montgomery AIDS Outreach Inc.
2900 McGeeHee Road
Montgomery, AL 36111
Phone: (334) 280-3349
www.maoi.org

GEORGIA

AID Atlanta
1605 Peachtree Street NE
Atlanta, GA 30309
Phone: (404) 870-7720

Fax: (404) 870-7719

www.aidatlanta.org

FLORIDA

**Okaloosa AIDS Support and
Informational Services, Inc. (OASIS)**

745 NW Beal Parkway, Suite 10

Fort Walton Beach, FL 32547

Phone: (850) 314-0950

Fax: (850) 314-0952

E-mail: aidsoasis1@aol.com

UF Rainbow Center at Shands Jacksonville

Clinical Center, Third Floor

655 W. Eighth Street

Jacksonville, FL 32209

Phone: (904) 244-3051

www.hscj.ufl.edu/rainbow

KENTUCKY

Matthew 25 AIDS Services, Inc.

452 Old Corydon Road

Henderson, KY 42420

Phone: (270) 826-0200

www.matthew25clinic.org

LOUISIANA

NO/AIDS Task Force

2601 Tulane Avenue, #500

New Orleans, LA 70119

Phone: (504) 821-2601, ext. 228

www.noaidstaskforce.org

Acadiana C.A.R.E.S.
203 West 3rd Street
Lafayette, LA 70501
Phone: (337) 233-2437, ext. 25
www.acadianacares.com

MARYLAND

Sisters Together and Reaching, Inc. (STAR)
1505 Eutaw Place
Baltimore, MD 21217
Phone: (410) 383-1903
Fax: (410) 383-7856
www.sisterstogetherandreaching.org

NORTH CAROLINA

Alliance of AIDS Services Carolina
P.O. Box 12583
Raleigh, NC 27605
Phone: (919) 834-2437
Fax: (919) 834-3404
www.aas-c.org

RAIN Inc. (Regional AIDS Interfaith Network)
First United Methodist Church
501 North Tryon Street 4th Floor
Charlotte, NC 28202
Phone: (704) 372-7246
Fax: (704) 372-7418
www.carolinarain.org/home

OKLAHOMA

AIDS Walk of OKC, Inc.
1520 N. Robinson Avenue

Oklahoma City, OK 73103
Phone: (405) 525-2226
www.aidswalkokc.org

SOUTH CAROLINA

Catawba Care, Christopher Clinic
500 Lakeshore Parkway
Rock Hill, SC 29730
Phone: (803) 909-6363
www.catawbacare.org

S.C. HIV/AIDS Care Crisis Task Force
P.O. Box 2513
Columbia, SC 29202
Phone: (803) 254-6644

SC HIV AIDS Council
1115 Calhoun Street
Columbia, SC 29201
Phone: (803) 254-6644
www.schivaidscouncil.org

TENNESSEE

Nashville CARES
501 Brick Church Park Drive
Nashville, TN 37207-3219
Phone: (615) 259-4866, ext. 215
www.nashvillecares.org

TEXAS

Legacy Community Health
1116 Jackson Boulevard
Houston, TX 77006

Phone: (713) 830-3038
www.legacycommunityhealth.org

Resource Center Dallas
John Thomas Gay & Lesbian Community Center offices
2701 Reagan Street (at Brown)
Dallas, TX 75219
Phone: (214) 528-0144 or (866) 657-AIDS [(866) 657-2437]
www.rcdallas.org

International AIDS Empowerment
800 Montana Avenue
El Paso, TX 79902
Phone: (915) 590-2118 or (888) 767-8474
www.internationalaids.org

WEST VIRGINIA

HIV Care Consortium
P.O. Box 6360
Wheeling, WV 26003-0805

Charleston AIDS Network
Charleston, WV 25324
Phone: (304) 345-4673
E-mail: can@aidsnet.net
www.aidsnet.net

STATE HEALTH CARE AGENCIES

Alabama Department of Public Health
The RSA Tower, Suite 1400
P.O. Box 303017
Montgomery, AL 36130-3017
Phone: (334) 206-5364 or (800) ALA-1818
www.adph.org

Arkansas Department of Health
4815 West Markham Street
Little Rock, AR 72205
Phone: (501) 661-2000 or (800) 462-0599
www.healthyarkansas.gov

District of Columbia Department of Health
899 North Capitol Street NE
Washington, DC 20002
Phone: (202) 442 5955
http://doh.dc.gov/doh/site/default.asp

Delaware Division of Public Health
417 Federal Street, #1
Dover, DE 19901
Phone: (302) 744-4700
www.dhss.delaware.gov/dph

Florida Department of Health
2585 Merchants Row Boulevard
Tallahassee, FL 32311
Phone: (850) 245-4444
www.doh.state.fl.us

Georgia Division of Public Health
Georgia HIV Unit
#2 Peachtree Street, 12th Floor
Atlanta, GA 30303
Phone: (404) 657-3100
http://health.state.ga.us/programs/stdhiv

Kentucky Department for Public Health
275 East Main Street
Mail Stop HS 2EC
Frankfort, KY 40621-0001

Phone: (502) 564-6539, ext. 3552, or (800) 420-7431
http://chfs.ky.gov/dph

Louisiana Department of Health and Hospitals
Office of Public Health
28 N. 4th Street
Baton Rouge, LA 70802
Phone: (225) 342-9500
http://new.dhh.louisiana.gov

Maryland Department of Health and Mental Hygiene
500 N. Calvert Street
Baltimore, MD 21202
Phone: (410) 767-5013
http://dhmh.md.gov

Mississippi Department of Health
570 E. Woodrow Wilson Boulevard
Jackson, MS 39215-1700
Phone: (601) 576-7723
www.msdh.state.ms.us/index.htm

North Carolina Division of Public Health
1902 Mail Service Center
Raleigh, NC 27576
Phone: (919) 733-7301
http://publichealth.nc.gov/index.htm

Oklahoma Department of Health
1000 NE 10th
Oklahoma City, OK 73117
Phone: (405) 271-5600 or (800) 522-0203
www.ok.gov/health/index.html

South Carolina Department of Health and Environmental Control
2600 Bull Street
Columbia, SC 29201
Phone: (803) 898-DHEC [898-3432]
www.dhec.sc.gov

Tennessee Department of Health
Cordell Hull Building, 4th Floor
425 5th Avenue N
Nashville, TN 37247-4911
Phone: (615) 532-7188
http://health.state.tn.us/index.htm

Texas Department of State Health Services
4110 Guadalupe Building 636
Austin, TX 78751
Phone: (512) 533-3000
Fax: (512) 371-4672
www.dshs.state.tx.us/hivstd/default.shtm

Virginia Department of Health
109 Governor Street
Richmond, VA 23219
Phone: (804) 864-7955
www.vdh.state.va.us

West Virginia Department of Health and Human Resources
State Capitol Complex, Building 3, Room 206
Charleston, WV 25305
Phone: (304) 558-0684
www.wvdhhr.org

NATIONAL AIDS ORGANIZATIONS

The AIDS Institute
1705 DeSales Street NW, Suite 700
Washington, DC 20036
Phone: (202) 835-8373
www.theaidsinstitute.org

AIDS Action
1730 M Street NW, Suite 611
Washington, DC 20036
Phone: (202) 530-8030
Fax: (202) 530-8031
www.aac.org

Black AIDS Institute
1833 West 8th Street, Suite 200
Los Angeles, CA 90057
Phone: (213) 353-3610
Fax: (213) 989-0181
www.blackaids.org

American Foundation for AIDS Research (amfAR)
120 Wall Street, 13th Floor
New York, NY 10005-3902
Phone: (212) 806-1600 or (800) 392-6327
www.amfar.org

INFORMATIONAL AIDS WEBSITES

US National Library of Medicine (NLM) MEDLINEplus
This includes information from the National Institutes of Health and other government sources on over five hundred diseases and conditions. It also includes lists of hospitals and physicians, a medical encyclopedia and dictionaries, health information in Spanish, extensive information on prescrip-

tion and nonprescription drugs, health information from the media, and links to thousands of clinical trials.
www.nlm.nih.gov/medlineplus

AEGIS: AIDS Education Global Information System

This provides access to the latest news on HIV and AIDS, HIV-related articles from major wire services and newspapers across the United States, an extensive online library of HIV/AIDS-related journals, and a database of scientific abstracts and other related documents. It is fully indexed and searchable.
www.aegis.com

AIDS Action

AIDS Action is a national AIDS advocacy and public policy organization. Its Web site provides comprehensive policy and legislative advocacy resources and information related to AIDS funding appropriations, health care/treatment access, housing, prevention, research, and the Ryan White CARE Act. The site also features State of AIDS Online Discussion Board.
www.aidsaction.org

AIDS Housing of Washington

AIDS Housing of Washington is a Seattle-based nonprofit that develops HIV/AIDS housing locally and provides technical assistance nationally.
www.aidshousing.org

Healthology: HIV and AIDS

Healthology provides information and articles targeted to people living with HIV/AIDS. Topics are current and extensive and focus on health, treatment, and daily living.
http://nmac.healthology.com/focus_index

HIV Glossary

This is a compilation of definitions for words commonly used to describe HIV, associated treatments, and the medical management of related conditions.
www.aidsinfo.nih.gov/ed_resources/gov

HIV InSite

HIV InSite is a project of the University of California, San Francisco AIDS Research Institute, the AIDS Program at San Francisco General Hospital, the Center for AIDS Prevention Studies, and the Henry J. Kaiser Family Foundation. This website features information on medical research, prevention and education, social issues, and community resources.
http://hivinsite.ucsf.edu/InSite

HIV/AIDS Law and Police Resource

This is a destination for accurate, authoritative information on HIV law and policy issues. It includes contents of the publication *AIDS and the Law* (3rd edition), authored by David Webber, who created this website.
www.aidsandthelaw.com

Kaiser Family Foundation: HIV/AIDS Data and Statistics

This site is a gateway to HIV/AIDS statistics and key data available from the Kaiser Family Foundation, including links to HIV/AIDS fact sheets and state-by-state AIDS and other health-related data.
www.kff.org/hivaids/reporting/data

National AIDS Fund

This is one of America's largest philanthropic organizations dedicated to eliminating HIV/AIDS as a major health and social problem. The site includes information on workplace resources and a section about the Return-to-Work Initiative, which lists links to helpful articles, charts, and interviews.
www.nationalaidsfund.org

National Association of People with AIDS (NAPWA)

NAPWA's website features information about program activities—including AIDSWATCH—news and bulletins, and access to NAPWA newsletters and publications, conference announcements, and other HIV/AIDS-related resources.
www.napwa.org

National Minority AIDS Council (NMAC)

This national AIDS organization develops programs and services for community-based organizations serving people of color affected by HIV/AIDS. The website provides information about NMAC conferences (including the US Conference on AIDS), public policy efforts, research and treatment advocacy programs, technical assistance activities, and publications.
www.nmac.org

National AIDS Treatment Advocacy Project (NATAP)

The National AIDS Treatment Advocacy Project tries to facilitate the development of effective treatment for HIV by advocating on treatment and policy issues for people with HIV and AIDS with drug companies and government officials.
www.natap.org

Phoenix Rising HIV/AIDS Re-entry Project

This is an online guide designed to foster independence, empowerment, and self-sufficiency for people living with AIDS. Topics include planning for work and school, laws, benefits and work, and money management.
www.phoenixrisingreentry.org

Project Inform

Project Inform is a national, nonprofit, community-based organization that seeks to end the AIDS epidemic. It provides free, confidential, and empowering information. The site includes publications, outreach and education, advocacy programs related to AIDS/HIV, and a national HIV/AIDS treatment hotline.
www.projectinform.org

TA Clearinghouse

The TA Clearinghouse website is a news service for New York City community-based AIDS organizations, hosted by Bailey House, Inc., a nonprofit AIDS housing and service organization. The TA Clearinghouse provides searchable databases of the New York area technical assistance providers, funding alerts for HIV/AIDS service organizations, and a job bank.
www.taclearinghouse.org

The Body

The Body is a "multimedia AIDS and HIV information resource" focusing on treatment, legal, mental health, and political issues and providing a way for people to connect with one another on the website through forums and direct contact with the organizations listed. The site includes access to AIDS Action, AIDS National Interfaith Network, amfAR, American Psychiatric Association, Gay Men's Health Crisis, Johns Hopkins University AIDS Service, Lambda Legal Defense and Treatment Action Group, and the National Minority AIDS Council.
www.thebody.com

National Prevention Information Network (NPIN)

The CDC's NPIN is the US reference and referral service for information on HIV/AIDS, viral hepatitis, sexually transmitted diseases (STDs), and tuberculosis. NPIN produces, collects, catalogs, and electronically disseminates materials and information to organizations and people working in those disease fields in national, state, and local settings. NPIN also manages www.hivtest.org, the national HIV and STD testing site locator service. Call (800) 458-5231.
www.cdcnpin.org and www.hivtest.org

American Academy of HIV Medicine

This is an independent organization of HIV specialists and others dedicated to promoting excellence in HIV/AIDS care. Using advocacy and education, the Academy supports health care providers in HIV medicine and works to ensure better care for those living with HIV and AIDS. Call (202) 659-0699. www.aahivm.org.

Family Health International

Family Health International (FHI) is among the largest and most established nonprofit organizations actively dedicated to improving the lives of people with HIV/AIDS worldwide through research, education, and services in family health. The organization focuses on developing strategies to respond to the HIV/AIDS pandemic, other sexually transmitted

infections, and unintended pregnancies. Location: Research Triangle Park, NC. Call (919) 544-7040.
www.fhi.org/en/index.htm

Gay Men's Health Crisis (GMHC)
GMHC offers a hotline, counseling, and workshop information on the basics on AIDS, HIV testing, safer sex, caring for yourself and your friends, and useful facts and newsletters. Educational materials, booklets, brochures, videos, manuals, posters, buttons, newsletters, condoms, and more are available.
www.gmhc.org

Health Resources and Services Administration (HRSA) HIV/AIDS Programs
The HRSA HIV/AIDS Bureau, one of four bureaus of the Health Resources and Services Administration, is the largest single source, next to the Medicaid and Medicare programs, of federal funding for HIV/AIDS care for low-income individuals.
http://hab.hrsa.gov

AIDS Vaccine Advocacy Coalition (AVAC)
AVAC is a community- and consumer-based organization, founded in December 1995, to accelerate the ethical development and global delivery of vaccines against HIV/AIDS. It provides independent analysis, policy advocacy, public education, and mobilization to enhance AIDS vaccine research and development.
www.avac.org

National Institutes of Health (NIH)
The NIH is one of the world's foremost biomedical research centers and the federal focal point for biomedical research in the United States.
www.nih.gov

AIDS Clinical Trials Group (ACTG)
ACTG, the largest HIV clinical trials organization in the world, plays a major role in setting standards of care for HIV infection and opportunistic

diseases related to HIV/AIDS in the United States and the developed world.

https://actgnetwork.org

AIDSinfo (NIH)

AIDSinfo is a central resource for current information on federally and privately funded clinical trials for AIDS patients and others infected with HIV. This is the main dissemination point for federally approved HIV treatment and prevention guidelines. AIDSinfo also provides information about treatment regimens for HIV infection and AIDS-related illnesses, including the prevention of HIV transmission from occupational exposure and mother-to-child transmission during pregnancy.

http://aidsinfo.nih.gov

AIDS Research Institute at University of California San Francisco (UCSF)

UCSF provides links to programs including clinical and research studies, virology programs, clinical trials, and others.

http://ari.ucsf.edu

American Social Health Association (ASHA)

ASHA's mission is to stop sexually transmitted diseases and their harmful consequences to individuals, families, and communities. It produces information on HIV/AIDS and STDs including educational materials, newsletters, and other resources.

www.ashastd.org

Centers for Disease Control and Prevention (CDC)

The CDC website covers a wide range of HIV/AIDS topics including basic science, surveillance, prevention tools, training tools, basic statistics, brochures, fact sheets, slide sets, conference updates, and other relevant information.

www.cdc.gov

Journal of the American Medical Association (*JAMA*): HIV/AIDS Resource Center

JAMA's HIV/AIDS Resource Center is an interactive collection of resources for physicians, other health professionals, and the public. Included are links to clinical updates, news, and information on a broad range of social and policy questions relating to HIV/AIDS.

http://jama.ama-assn.org

AIDS Healthcare Foundation

Los Angeles–based AIDS Healthcare Foundation (AHF) is a global organization providing cutting-edge medicine and advocacy to over 100,000 people in twenty-two countries. It is the nation's largest provider of HIV/AIDS medical care.

www.aidshealth.org

Immunization Action Coalition (IAC)

This site offers patient and physician information on hepatitis A and B. Includes downloadable brochures, *Needle Tips* newsletter, guidelines, and fact sheets in English, Spanish, Chinese, Vietnamese, Farsi, Tagalog, Cambodian, Russian, Korean, Hmong, and Laotian and information on vaccination schedules, risk factors, and universal precautions. IAC has over a dozen educational videos, some for providers and more for patients. Seven are in languages other than English.

www.immunize.org

US Department of Health and Human Services (HHS)

HHS provides many programs that deal with AIDS and other health issues.

www.hhs.gov

US Food and Drug Administration (FDA)

The FDA homepage includes news and information on foods, human drugs, biologics, medical devices and radiological health, toxicology, and more.

www.fda.gov

HIV/AIDS/STD CLINICAL AND TREATMENT RESOURCES

National Network of STD/HIV Prevention Training Centers
The National Network of STD/HIV Prevention Training Centers is a group of regional centers created to increase the knowledge and skills of health care professionals in the area of sexual and reproductive health.
http://depts.washington.edu/nnptc

National AIDS Treatment Advocacy Project (NATAP)
NATAP facilitates efforts for the development of effective treatment for HIV by advocating on treatment and policy issues for people with HIV and AIDS with drug companies, government officials (including FDA), and other treatment and policy advocates.
http://depts.washington.edu/nnptc

The Gay And Lesbian National Hotline (GLBT National Help Center)
The Gay and Lesbian National Hotline is a nonprofit, tax-exempt organization dedicated to meeting the needs of the gay and lesbian community by offering free and totally anonymous information, referrals, and peer counseling. Callers speak to a trained volunteer who will be able to access a national database of referrals specific to the gay and lesbian community.
(888) THE-GLNH [843-4564]
Hours: Monday–Friday, 4 PM to midnight ET; Saturday noon to 5 PM ET
www.glnh.org

The White House Office of National AIDS Policy
The Office of National AIDS Policy coordinates the administration's domestic efforts to reduce the number of new HIV and AIDS infections in the United States, in particular in segments of the population that are experiencing new or renewed increases in the rate of infection.
(202) 456-7320
www.whitehouse.gov/onap/aids

INTERNATIONAL ORGANIZATIONS

World Health Organization (WHO)

The WHO HIV/AIDS Department provides "evidence based" technical support to member states to help them deal with treatment, care, prevention services, and drug and diagnostics supply to ensure a sustainable response to HIV/AIDS. Based in Geneva, Switzerland, the agency is a cosponsor of UNAIDS.

Email: hiv-aids@who.int
www.who.int/hiv/en/

UNAIDS

The Joint United Nations Programme on AIDS/HIV has a vision of zero deaths, zero discrimination, and zero new infections from HIV/AIDS. The agency, which has a secretariat in Geneva, Switzerland, and seven regional offices, tries to promote global access to HIV prevention, care, treatment, and support.

www.unaids.org/eng/

SOURCES

This work began as a simple idea: what if I wrote a book about the story of AIDS in Clover? What followed were countless hours of telephone interviews with Reverend Patricia Ann Starr and others from 2005 to 2010. In researching and writing this book I have drawn heavily from my previous columns written for the *Rock Hill* (South Carolina) *Herald*, personal recollections, and a wide array of public sources.

Because notes can distract the reader I have avoided using them in the text. I have quoted directly from sources using quotation marks and have paraphrased in other places.

Prologue

"HIV/AIDS and Other Sexually Transmitted Diseases (STDs) in the Southern Region of the United States: An Epidemiological Overview." Kaiser Family Foundation website, November 13, 2002. www.kff.org /hivaids/6062-index.cfm.

Chapter 1: The Final Call

The Southern States Manifesto: HIV/AIDS and STDs in the South: A Call to Action. Southern States AIDS/STD Directors Work Group, March 2, 2003. www.southernaidscoalition.org/policy/SouthernStatesManifesto_2003.pdf.

The Southern States Manifesto:Update 2008, HIV/AIDS and Sexually Transmitted Diseases in the South. Southern States AIDS/STD Directors Work Group. www.southernaidscoalition.org/policy.html.

Southern States Summit on HIV/AIDS and STDs. November 13, 2002. www.kff.org/hivaids/20021113a-index.cfm.

"Growing HIV/AIDS Crisis in the South to Be Tackled by New Initiative." National AIDS Fund press release. September 28, 2007.

CDC AIDS surveillance and history.
www.cdc.gov/hiv/topics/surveillance/resources/reports/past.htm#su.

Chapter 2: Carolyn
Lyndon B. Johnson's 1964 State of the Union speech, January 8, 1964.
www.C-Span.org.

Clover History: Town of Clover website. www.cloversc.info.

First Baptist Church of Clover website. http://firstbaptistclover.org.

Chapter 5: Bad Blood
"Conference on Preventing Disease/Promoting Health—Objectives for the
Nation: Sexually Transmissible Diseases." *Sexually Transmitted Diseases* vol.
6, issue 4. October/December 1979. 272–277.

Robert B. Stroube, MD. "Infectious Syphilis Epidemic: Disease Control in the
United States: A Historical Overview." *Infectious Diseases.* May 2008. 68–70.

Peterman, T., Heffelfinger, J., Swint, E., et al. "The Changing Epidemiol-
ogy of Syphilis." *Sexually Transmitted Diseases.* 2005. 32 (suppl): S4–S10.

"The National Plan to Eliminate Syphilis from the United States." Atlanta:
US Department of Health and Human Services, Centers for Disease Control
and Prevention (CDC). May 8, 2006. www.cdc.gov/stdconference/2006
/media/SEE-fact-sheet.htm.

Lou Cannon. "President Reagan: The Role of a Lifetime" *Public Affairs.*
2000.

Centers for Diseases Control and Prevention. "Pneumocystis Pneumonia—
Los Angeles," *Morbidity and Mortality Weekly Report,* June 5, 1981. www
.cdc.gov/mmwr/preview/mmwrhtml/june_5.htm.

Chapter 6: The AIDS Doctor
Medical University of South Carolina history: www.musc.edu.

Alabama Department of Archives and History. www.archives.state.al.us.

Centers for Diseases Control and Prevention. "Pneumocystis Pneumonia—Los Angeles," *Morbidity and Mortality Weekly Report,* June 5, 1981. www.cdc.gov/mmwr/preview/mmwrhtml/june_5.htm.

Chapter 16: Sandy
"Holding AIDS at Bay, Only to Face 'Lazarus Syndrome.'" *New York Times.* October 6, 1998.

Chapter 18: Moving On
US Department of Health and Human Services Health Resources and Services Administration HIV/AID Program. Ryan White CARE Act grants. http://hab.hrsa.gov.

Chapter 21: Carolyn: The Final Years
SC Senate Resolution S1148 by Sen. John Wesley Matthews Jr. March 21, 2002. www.scstatehouse.gov.

Chapter 23: A Call to Action
Southern States Summit on HIV/AIDS and STDs. November 13–15, 2002. Kaiser Family Foundation. www.kff.org/hivaids/20021113a-index.cfm.

Southern States Manifesto: A Call to Action. 2002. www.southernaidscoalition.org/policy/SouthernStatesManifesto_2003.pdf.

"HIV Clinic Spreading Word About Services." *Rock Hill Herald.* October 5, 2005.

"Fighting the AIDS Epidemic of Today: Reauthorizing the Ryan White CARE Act." US Senate Health, Education, Labor, and Pensions Committee Hearing, March 1, 2006. help.senate.gov/hearings/index.cfm?year=2006&month=03.

"HIV/AIDS in America: The Rural vs. Urban Funding Debate." *Congressional Digest.* December 2006, Vol. 85, No. 10.

INDEX

Acyclovir, 68, 70
African American AIDS funerals, 165–66
African Americans
  AIDS and, 8–10, 54, 196–97, 202, 241
  STDs and, 8–10, 52, 54–55, 66, 196–97,
    202, 241
AIDS (acquired immune deficiency syn-
    drome). *See also* HIV; *specific persons
    with AIDS*
  African Americans and, 8–10, 54, 196–
    97, 202, 241
  antiretroviral therapy for, 90, 95, 135,
    243–44, 272
  calculus of, 161
  confidentiality and, 80, 103–4, 121
  contagion of, 71, 80–82, 103
  demographics of, 8–11, 241
  denial of. *See* denial
  funding for, 9, 160, 233–35, 234, 241–45
  gays and, 10, 54–59, 65, 67–71, 81, 110
  grieving and, 79, 104, 107, 109–10, 159
  heterosexuals and, 8, 68–69, 202
  history of, 10, 58–59
  immune system and, 68
  intravenous drug use and, 8, 57, 69, 89,
    111
  living with relative dying of, 220
  medical workers' fear of, 80–81
  mother-to-child transmission, 95
  naming of, 69
  navy testing for, 120
  notification of sexual partners, 90, 161
  patient privacy/confidentiality, 80, 103–4,
    121
  patients' reactions to, 196–98
  in prison system, 133–36
  progress in care and treatment of, 272–73
  religious conservatism and, 103

routine and language of, 3
shame and. *See* shame
South Carolina's response to, 101–12
Southern AIDS Summit call to action,
    233–35
stigma surrounding, 73, 79–80, 110, 197,
    253
suicide and, 88, 196, 202, 228
as symptom of social inequalities and
    racial/ethnic health disparities, 11
unprotected sex and, xii, 58, 212, 224,
    272
AIDS Alabama, 243
AIDS Drugs Assistance Program, 244
AIDS education and training, 103
AIDS Housing Coalition, 196
Alexander, Mervin, 139–40
Alexander's Barber Shop and Quick Stop,
    139–40
Althea (Samuel Pegram's mistress), 32–35
American Red Cross, 102–4
antibody-antigen testing, 70
anticommunism, 106
antiretroviral therapy, 90, 95, 135, 243–44,
    272
the Arcade, 122
Armstrong, Bernitha Ann "Nita"
  background of, 177–80
  death of, 189–90
  getting saved, 182–83
  Linda Ashley and, 185–86
  niece Jesse and, 184
  refusing AIDS medication, 185–90
  Tricia Ann Starr and, 180–82, 185–90
Armstrong, Dorothy, 177–79
Armstrong, Lilly, 177–78
Ashe, Arthur, 70, 102
Ashley, Harriette Harold, 148–51, 153